For Matthew

The Anatomy Companion: Muscles of the Upper & Lower Extremity
Second Edition 2019

Cover/Content/Illustrations/Design/Layout by Sean de Lima Thie, DC
Written and Illustrated by Sean de Lima Thiel, DC
Foreword by P. Bailey McBride, MD
Copy Edited by Craig Strukoff
All images and content are © 2019 Cortical Media Inc.

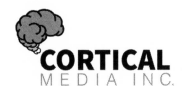

CORTICAL
M E D I A I N C.

All inquiries should be addressed to:

Cortical Media Inc.
www.corticalmedia.com ~ info.corticalmedia@gmail.com

ISBN:
9781698389899

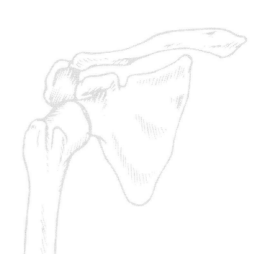

The Anatomy Companion:
Muscles of the
Upper & Lower
Extremities
Second Edition

Dr. Sean de Lima

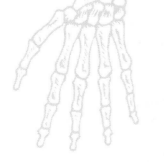

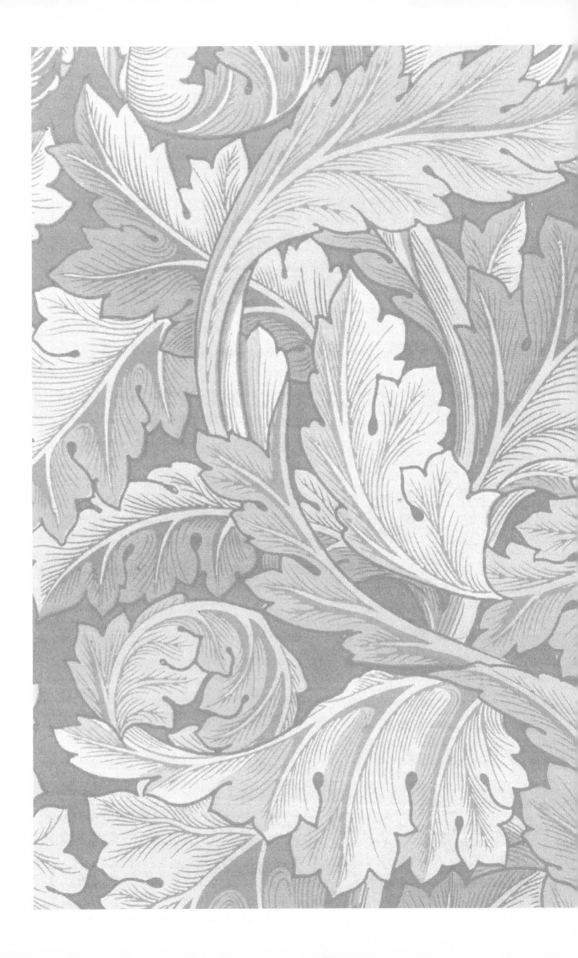

TABLE OF CONTENTS
Muscles of the Upper & Lower Extremities
Dr. Sean de Lima

FOREWORD
BY P. BAILEY MCBRIDE, MD

Anatomy is to the body what the alphabet is to reading. It is essential for success. "The Anatomy Companion" will help students learn to "read the body." For students in health-related studies, this book is the perfect companion to anatomy labs and serves as a supportive text for lecture material. Preparation for exams will never be easier. "The Anatomy Companion" is perfect for the student new to anatomy as well as a valuable resource for veteran anatomists looking for a concise review of human upper and lower extremity anatomy.

Anatomy has been a unifying theme for me and the author. In early years, I engaged in a formal program of study, graduating with a master's degree in Anatomy. I continued my passion for the study of the human body in medical school and went on to care for others through the practice of general surgery. Returning to higher education to share my enthusiasm for Anatomy as a professor at Life Chiropractic College West is both an honor and a delight. It is much like returning home. It is ever so familiar but continues to surprise me nonetheless.

One surprise was meeting Sean at Life Chiropractic College West. Sean has an unwavering thirst for knowledge combined with a skilled and generous approach to sharing it. He delivers uncommon value to those in his sphere. He galvanizes fellow students and mentors them through the learning process. This has given him a unique view of how students learn. That insight is evident in his current work. It is a book for students created by a student. Sean applies his professional artistic skills to the study of anatomical sciences. His artwork brings anatomy to life and his illustrations populate the work. "The Anatomy Companion" is exactly what is needed for the student to build a confident foundation in extremity anatomy.

The three parts of "The Anatomy Companion" combine anatomical accuracy with the learning power of imagination and the fun of a coloring book. Part I is organized by functional muscle groups of the upper and lower extremities. Illustrations are accompanied by descriptions of each muscle's origin, insertion, innervation, blood supply and function. In Part II, the student gets to apply their knowledge through coloring and labeling exercises. Labeling and quiz exercises reinforce the content ensuring an engaging and effective learning experience. Drawing exercises round out Part III to make this book a veritable learning trifecta. It showcases a hands-on learning approach created with the student in mind, front and center.

I only wish Sean had been in my anatomy class when I was a student and created such an extraordinary resource. It is an evergreen book that will be useful on your shelf for years to come serving as a quick reference. Like many great books, the worse it looks on your shelf from wear and tear, the better you look. I look forward to seeing more publications in the future that highlight Sean's anatomy and artistic superpowers.

P. Bailey McBride, MD

Acknowledgments

This book was inspired and made possible by
those who lead with passion and set a high standard for excellence.

Life Changing Teachers,

Thank you Baiely McBride, Sue Ray, Lauren Clum,
Ankur Tayal, Monique Andrews, Tamara MacIntyre, Mark Thompson, Norm Strutin,
Ramneek Bhogal, Stephanie O'Neill-Bhogal, and Barbara Delli Gatti.
The world need more minds like yours!

To Kevin Elander,

Thank you for helping me find the value of
understanding anatomy and its functional applications.

To Tyla Arnason & the Thrive Team,

Thank you for all the work that you do. Your commitment to health and
wellness was the initial spark that set me on the path to a career in healthcare.

INTRODUCTION
by Sean de Lima, DC

How To Use This Book:

I was introduced to clinical anatomy was during my under-graduate studies. My first anatomy course was held over twelve weeks, filled with countless hours of study and rote memorization.

Having a history in graphic design, it didn't take me long to recognize that I easily remembered a muscle's origins and insertions after I drew them. Using photocopies of skeletal arms or legs, I'd draw a muscle on each copy and label important information.

As a visual learner, I was happy to have found a remarkably successful study method!

By the time I completed that basic anatomy course, I had a series of drawings of most of the body's muscles. They were messy and had notes scribbled all over them. That was the first time I'd contemplated making an anatomy workbook.

Years later, during chiropractic college anatomy courses, I was astounded by the level of detail I could recall from my undergraduate muscle drawings. Again, the idea to produce an anatomy study tool popped into my head. In my spare time between classes, exams and homework, I researched and illustrated each of the muscles of the upper and lower extremities, compiling crucial information such as origins, insertions, blood supply, innervation and functions.

In making this book, I hope to create a valuable tool for anyone in health care or kineseology. This book is divided into three parts. Part I is a thorough and concise reference. Each muscle is presented individually to optimally highlight where it attaches. At the end of this section, labeled muscle groups will give you an idea of how each muscle is situated in relation to the others around it.

Part II offers coloring pages of each of the muscles. To the right of all the illustrations, you will have the opportunity to fill in important information (origin, insertion, innervation...). Come up with a color scheme that will work for you! Maybe all muscles of the radial nerve are shades of red and pank, while muscles of the median nerve are blue. Feel free to be creative here. The more fun you have when coloring these muscles, the better you will remember them!

Finally, Part III will cement your knowledge. There are pages with images of the skeletal structures and you get to draw the muscles yourself! You don't need to be an artist to benefit from this. By drawing, you are learning visually and kines-thetically at the same time.

To support your learning, you can visit www.corticalmeda.com to print off extra drawing pages to make travel flash-cards.

My hope is that this book not only helps you gain confidence in the field of anatomy, but helps you to find a deeper appreciation and understanding of how the body moves and functions. This book was created to be your go-to anatomy reference, your academic colleague and educational companion. The best way to show it love is to fill it with notes, doodles, drawings, coloring, questions, ideas and insights.

Good luck on your adventure into the world of anatomy. I hope you enjoy using this book as much as I enjoyed creating it!

~Sean de Lima, DC.

Part I is a thorough, and concise reference.
Each muscle is presented individually to optimally highlight
where it attaches to the skeleton. This book was created to be your go-to
anatomy resource, your academic colleague and companion. The best way to
show it love is to fill it with notes, doodles, drawings, coloring, questions, ideas
and insights. Don't be afraid to draw and write all over these pages!

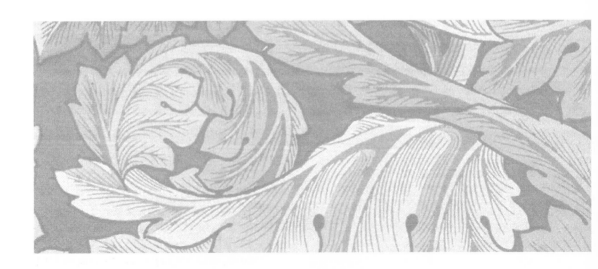

Part I:
Reference

Anterior Skeleton

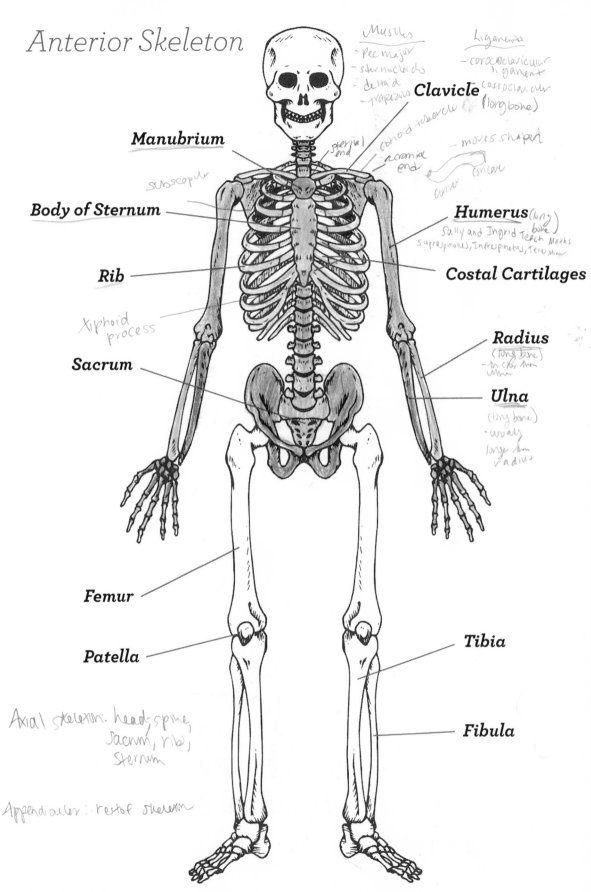

Clavicle

Manubrium

Body of Sternum

Rib

Sacrum

Femur

Patella

Humerus

Costal Cartilages

Radius

Ulna

Tibia

Fibula

Handwritten annotations:

Muscles
- Pec major
- sternocleido
- deltoid
- trapezius

Ligaments
- coracoclavicular ligament
costoclavicular (long bone)

cohoid tubercle

sternal end

acromial end

- moves shaped
Convex   Concave

subscapular

Humerus (long bone)
Sally and Ingrid Teach Maths
supraspinatus, Infraspinatus, Teres Minor

Radius (long bone)
- thicker than ulna

Ulna (long bone)
- usually longer than radius

xiphoid process

Axial skeleton: head, spine, sacrum, ribs, sternum

Appendicular: rest of skeleton

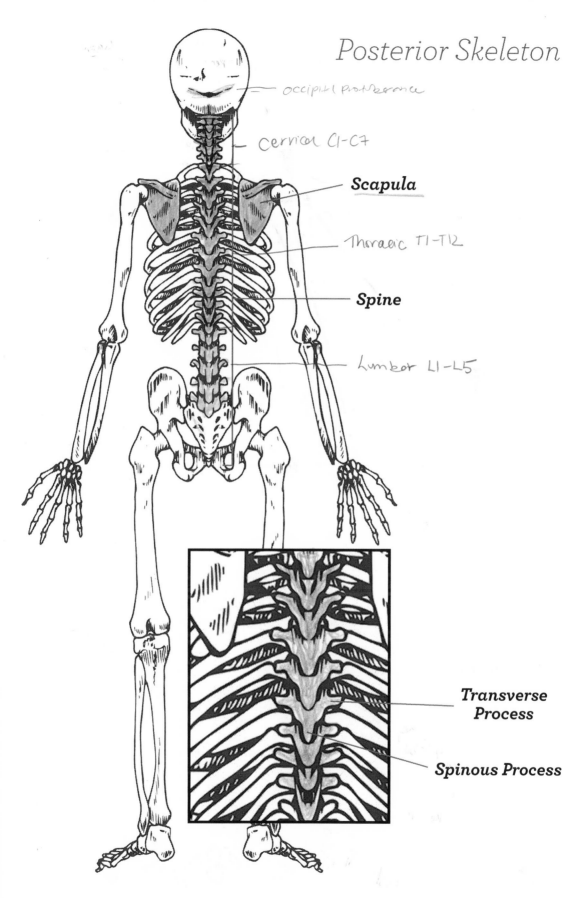

occipital protuberance

cervical C1-C7

Scapula

Thoracic T1-T12

Spine

Lumbar L1-L5

Transverse Process

Spinous Process

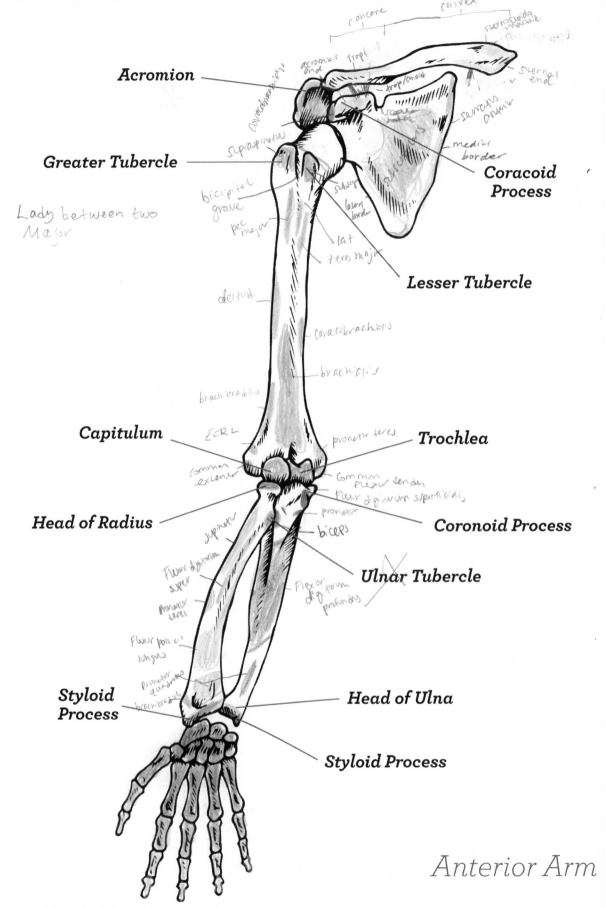

Acromion

Greater Tubercle

Lady between two Major

Capitulum

Head of Radius

Styloid Process

concave   convex

sternoclavicular joint (SC)

acromial end

trap'd

trap/onoid

scapular notch

subscapularis

medial border

Coracoid Process

coracobrachialis

supraspinatus

bicipital groove

pec major

subsc.

lesser border

lat

teres major

deltoid

coracobrachialis

brachialis

brachioradialis

ECRL

common extensor

pronator teres

common flexor tendon

flexor digitorum superficialis

pronator

supinator

Flexor digitorum super

pronator teres

Flexor pollicis longus

pronator quadratus

brachioradialis

Flexor digitorum profundus

biceps

serratus anterior

sternal end

Lesser Tubercle

Trochlea

Coronoid Process

Ulnar Tubercle

Head of Ulna

Styloid Process

Anterior Arm

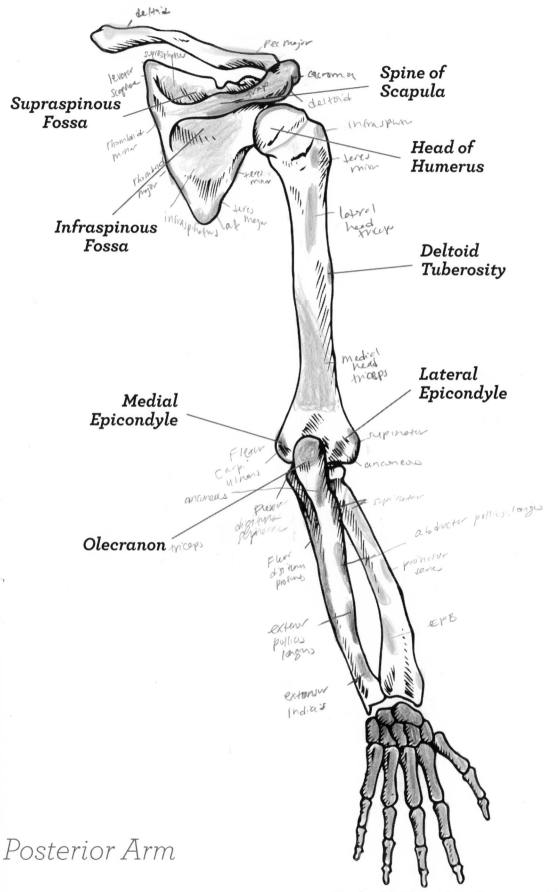

Supraspinous Fossa

Infraspinous Fossa

Spine of Scapula

Head of Humerus

Deltoid Tuberosity

Medial Epicondyle

Lateral Epicondyle

Olecranon

Posterior Arm

Hand, Palmar Aspect

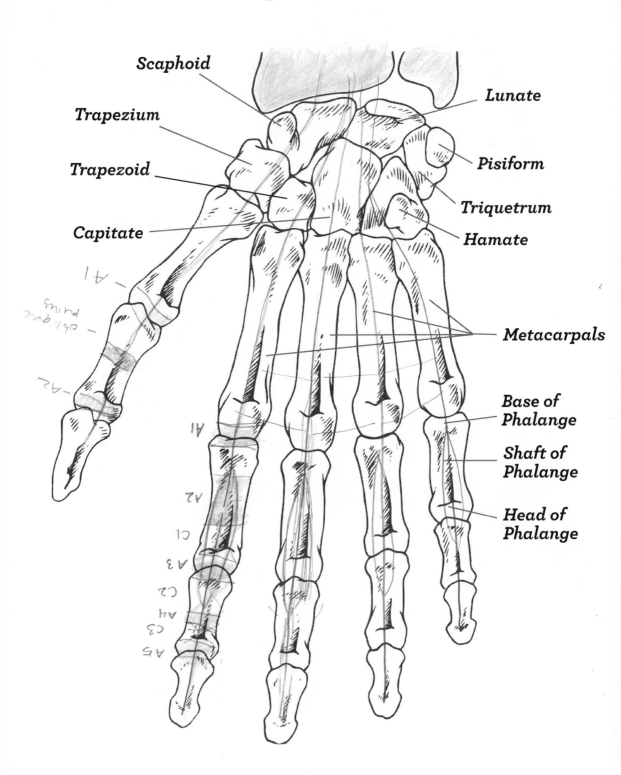

Scaphoid

Trapezium

Trapezoid

Capitate

Lunate

Pisiform

Triquetrum

Hamate

Metacarpals

Base of Phalange

Shaft of Phalange

Head of Phalange

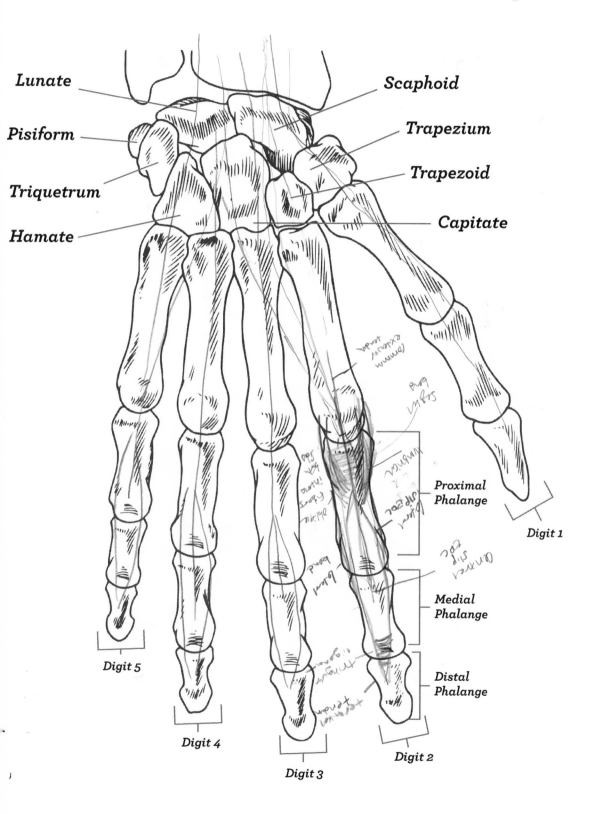

Lunate

Pisiform

Triquetrum

Hamate

Scaphoid

Trapezium

Trapezoid

Capitate

Proximal
Phalange

Digit 1

Medial
Phalange

Digit 5

Distal
Phalange

Digit 4

Digit 2

Digit 3

Anterior Leg

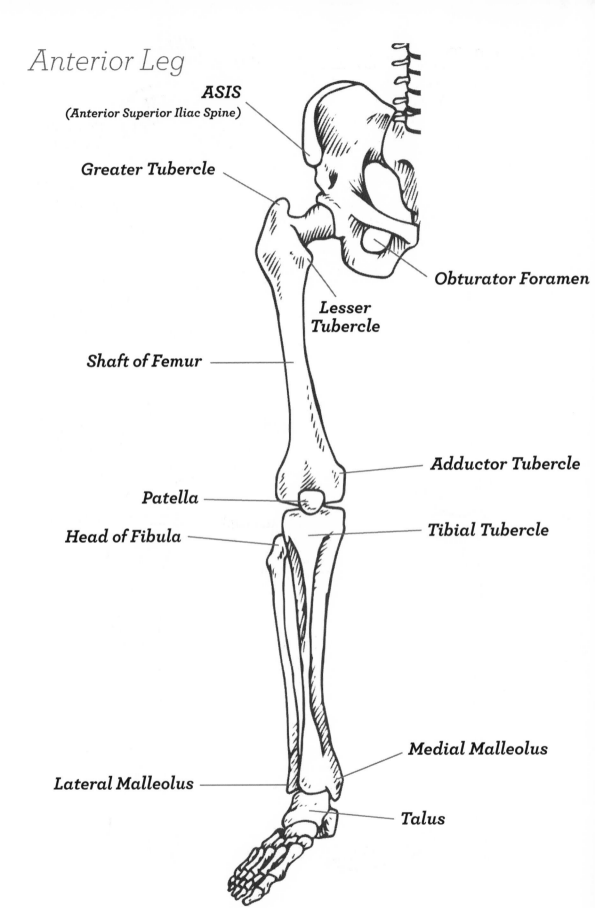

ASIS
(Anterior Superior Iliac Spine)

Greater Tubercle

Obturator Foramen

Lesser Tubercle

Shaft of Femur

Adductor Tubercle

Patella

Tibial Tubercle

Head of Fibula

Medial Malleolus

Lateral Malleolus

Talus

Lateral & Posterior Leg

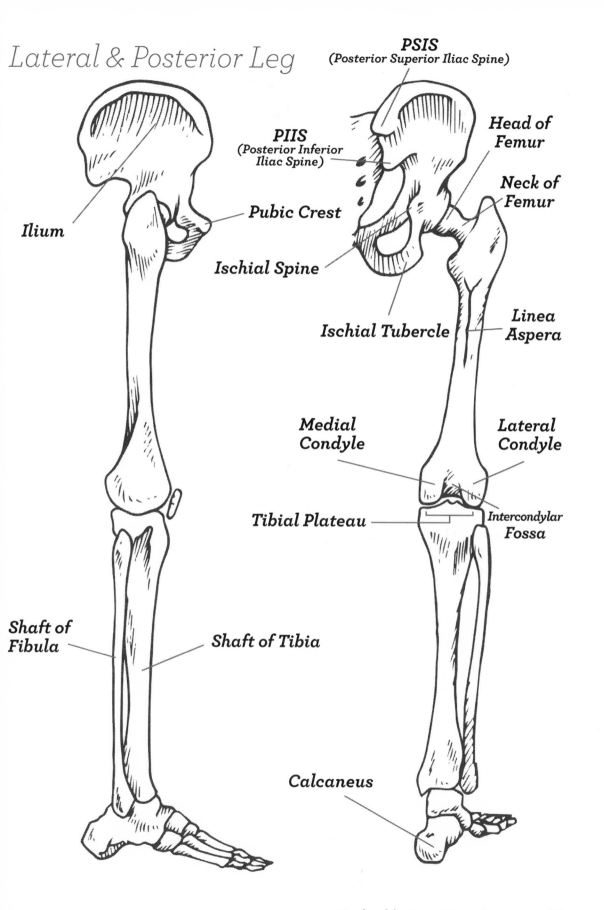

PSIS
(Posterior Superior Iliac Spine)

PIIS
(Posterior Inferior
Iliac Spine)

Head of
Femur

Neck of
Femur

Ilium

Pubic Crest

Ischial Spine

Ischial Tubercle

Linea
Aspera

Medial
Condyle

Lateral
Condyle

Tibial Plateau

Intercondylar
Fossa

Shaft of
Fibula

Shaft of Tibia

Calcaneus

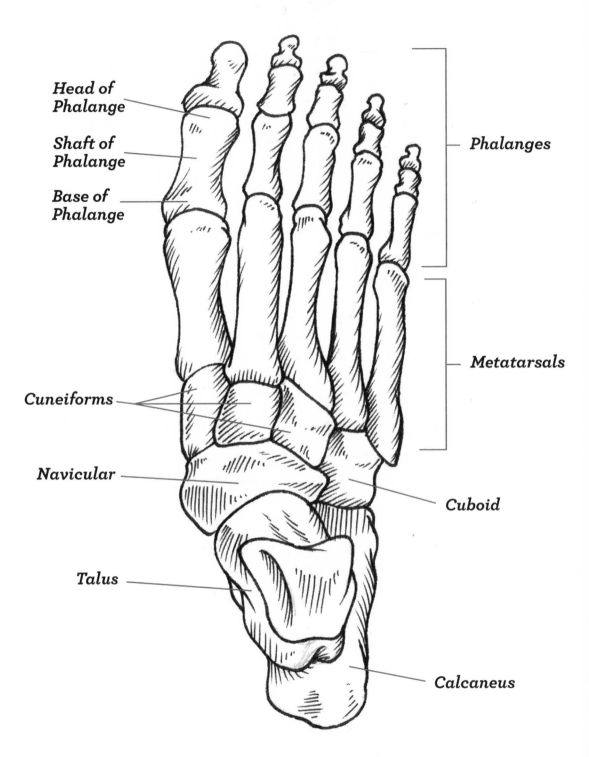

Head of
Phalange

Shaft of
Phalange

Base of
Phalange

Phalanges

Cuneiforms

Metatarsals

Navicular

Cuboid

Talus

Calcaneus

Foot, Dorsal Aspect

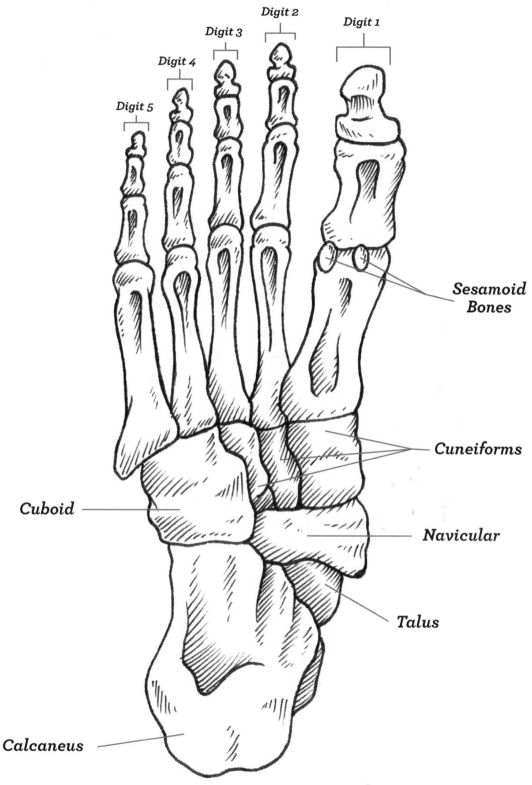

Digit 5

Digit 4

Digit 3

Digit 2

Digit 1

Sesamoid
Bones

Cuneiforms

Cuboid

Navicular

Talus

Calcaneus

Foot, Plantar Aspect

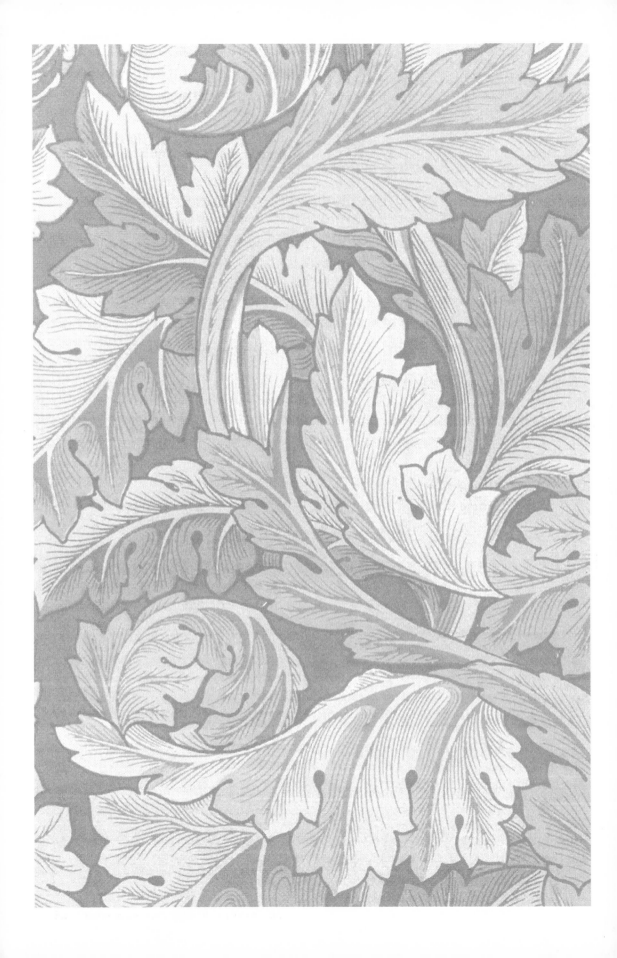

UPPER EXTREMITY

Brachial Plexus

The brachial plexus arises from the spinal cord in the cervical spine and carries commands from the brain to the muscles and other structures, and back from those structures to the brain. The combination of nerve roots form "terminal branches." Each branch has a unique name and supplies specific muscles.

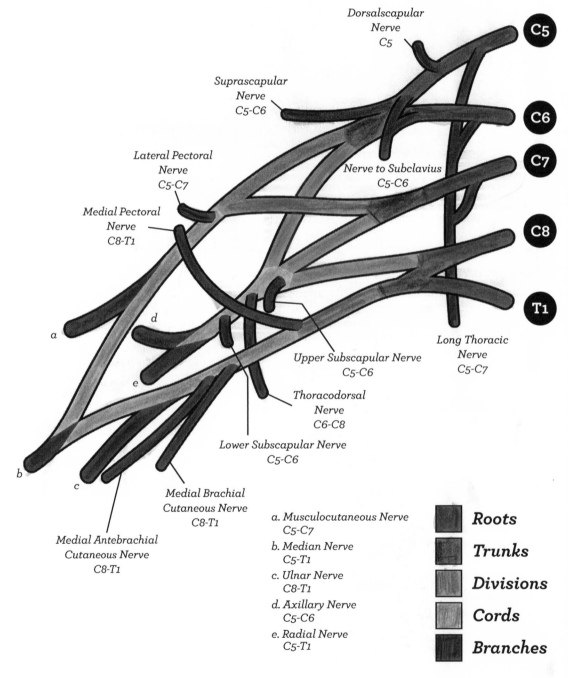

Dorsalscapular Nerve
C5

Suprascapular Nerve
C5-C6

Nerve to Subclavius
C5-C6

Lateral Pectoral Nerve
C5-C7

Medial Pectoral Nerve
C8-T1

C5

C6

C7

C8

T1

Long Thoracic Nerve
C5-C7

Upper Subscapular Nerve
C5-C6

Thoracodorsal Nerve
C6-C8

Lower Subscapular Nerve
C5-C6

Medial Brachial Cutaneous Nerve
C8-T1

Medial Antebrachial Cutaneous Nerve
C8-T1

a. Musculocutaneous Nerve
C5-C7
b. Median Nerve
C5-T1
c. Ulnar Nerve
C8-T1
d. Axillary Nerve
C5-C6
e. Radial Nerve
C5-T1

Roots

Trunks

Divisions

Cords

Branches

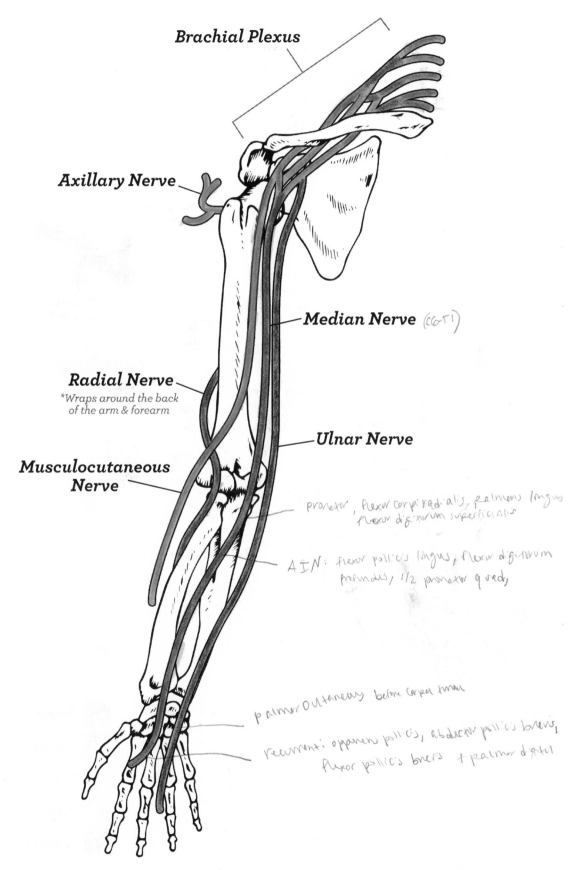

Brachial Plexus

Axillary Nerve

Median Nerve (C6-T1)

Radial Nerve
*Wraps around the back
of the arm & forearm*

Ulnar Nerve

**Musculocutaneous
Nerve**

pronator, flexor corpi radialis, palmaris longus
flexor digitorum superficialis

A I N: flexor pollicis longus, flexor digitorum
profundus, 1/2 pronator quad,

palmar cutaneous before carpal tunnel

recurrent: opponens pollicis, abductor pollicis brevis,
flexor pollicis brevis + palmar digital

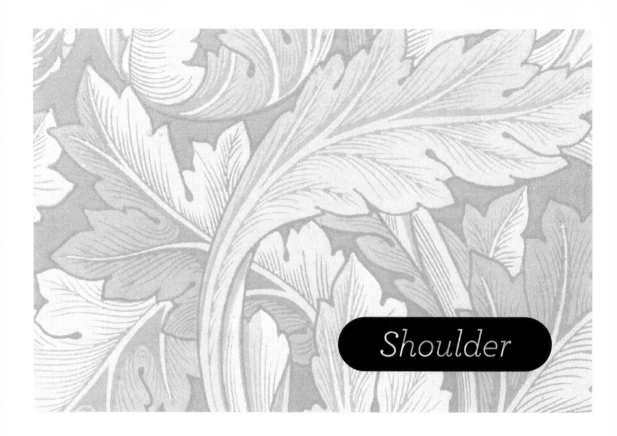

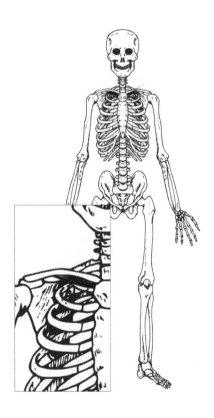

Subclavius

Origin:
Ventral Aspect Of Rib 1

Insertion:
Inferior Aspect Of Mid Clavicle

Innervation:
Nerve To Subclavius (C5-C6)

Blood Supply:
Pectoral Branch Of Thoracoacromial
Trunk

Function:
Assists In Rib Cage Elevation During Inspiration;
Draws Scapula Anterior And Inferior.

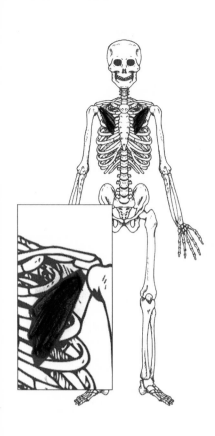

Pectoralis Minor

Origin:
Anterolateral Aspect Of Ribs 3-5,
Near The Costal Cartilage

Insertion:
Coracoid Process

Innervation:
Medial Pectoral Nerve (C8-T1)

Blood Supply:
Pectoral Branch Of Thoracoacromial
Trunk

Function:
*Rib Cage Elevation During Inspiration;
Scapula Protraction*

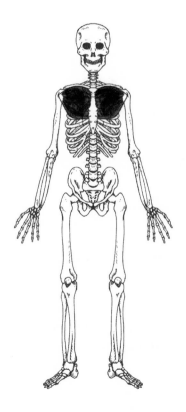

Pectoralis Major

Origin:
Clavicular Head– Ventral Aspect, Medial
Border Of Clavicle; *Sternocostal Head–*
Anterior Sternum, Upper 6 Costal Cartilages

Insertion:
Lateral Lip Of Bicipital Groove Of Humerus

Innervation:
Lateral Pectoral Nerve & Medial Pectoral
Nerve (Clavicular Head– C5-C7; Sternocos-
tal Head– C8-T1)

Blood Supply:
Pectoral Branch Of Thoracoacromial Trunk

Function:
*Humerus Internal Rotation, Adduction; Aids In
Shoulder Protraction*

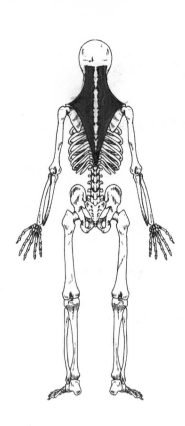

Trapezius

Origin:
External Occipital Protuberance, Superior
Nuchal Line, Spinous Processes Of C1-T12

Insertion:
Lateral Clavicle, Acromion Process,
Spine Of Scapula

Innervation:
CN XI & Ventral Rami (C3-C4)

Blood Supply:
Transverse Cervical

Function:
Upper Portion: Bilaterally= Extends Head And Neck,
Unilaterally= Laterally Flexes Head And Neck; Mid &
Lower Portions: Scapula Retraction And Depression

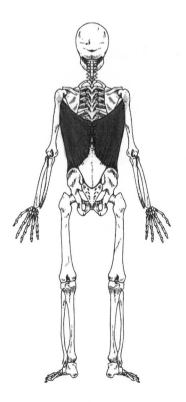

Latissimus Dorsi

Origin:
T7-T12 Spinous Processes & L1-L5
Spinous Processes Via The Lumbodorsal
Fascia, Iliac Crests, Lower 3 Ribs

Insertion:
Medial Lip Of Bicipital Groove Of Humerus

Innervation:
Thoracodorsal Nerve (C6-C8)

Blood Supply:
Thoracodorsal Artery

Function:
Brachium Internal Rotation, Extension, Adduction

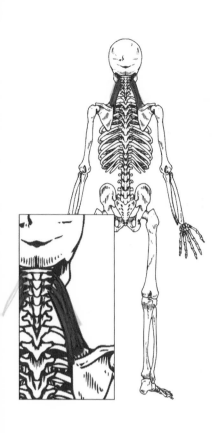

Levator Scapulae

Origin:
C1-C4 Transverse Processes

Insertion:
Medial Border, Superior Angle Of Scapula

Innervation:
Dorsal Scapular Nerve (C3-C5)

Blood Supply:
Deep Transverse Cervical Artery

Function:
Scapula Elevation; Neck Lateral Flexion

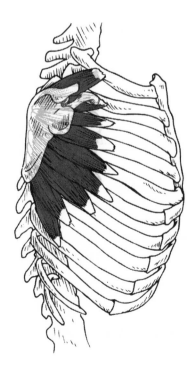

Serratus Anterior

Origin:
Lateral Aspect Of Ribs 1-9

Insertion:
Medial Border, Ventral Aspect
Of Scapula

Innervation:
Long Thoracic Nerve (C5-C7)

Blood Supply:
Lateral Thoracic Artery

Function:
Scapula Protraction; Rib Elevation

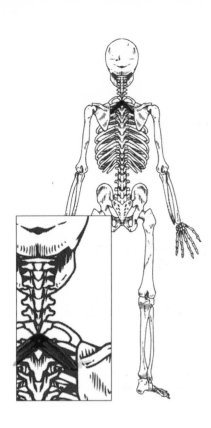

Rhomboid Minor

Origin:
 C7-T1 Spinous Processes

Insertion:
 Medial Border, Scapula At Base Of
 Scapular Spine

Innervation:
 Dorsal Scapular Nerve (C5)

Blood Supply:
 Dorsal Scapular Artery

Function:
 Scapula Elevation, Retraction, Rotation
 (Inferior Angle Toward Spine)

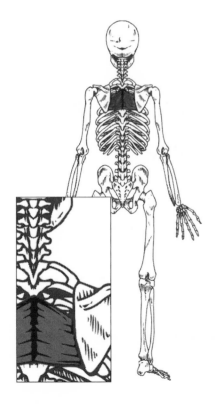

Rhomboid Major

Origin:
 T2-T5 Spinous Processes

Insertion:
 Medial Border Of Scapula

Innervation:
 Dorsal Scapular Nerve (C5)

Blood Supply:
 Dorsal Scapular Artery

Function:
 Scapula Elevation, Retraction, Rotation (Inferior
 Angle Toward Spine)

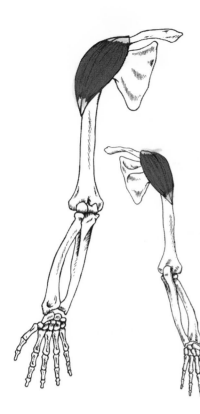

Deltoid

Origin:
Anterior Head– Lateral Clavicle; *Medial Head*– Acromion Process; *Posterior Head*– Lateral Spine Of Scapula

Insertion:
Deltoid Tuberosity Of Humerus

Innervation:
Axillary Nerve– Anterior And Posterior Circumflex Branches (C5-C6)

Blood Supply:
Thoracoacromial Artery And Branches Of Humeral Circumflex Artery

Function:
Medial Head– Humerus Abduction; Anterior Head– Humerus Flexion; Posterior Head–Humerus Extension

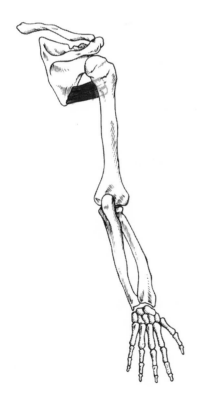

Teres Major

Origin:
Dorsal Aspect, Inferior Angle Of Scapula

Insertion:
Medial Lip Of Bicipital Groove Of Humerus

Innervation:
Lower Subscapular Nerve (C5-C6)

Blood Supply:
Posterior Humeral & Thoracodorsal Artery

Function:
Brachium Internal Rotation, Extension, Adduction

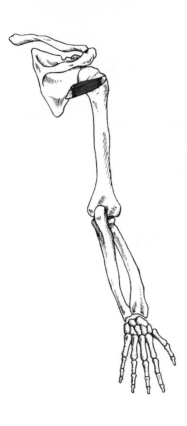

Teres Minor

Origin:
Dorsal Aspect, Axillary Border Of Scapula

Insertion:
Inferior Dorsal Aspect Of Greater Tuberosity Of Humerus (Partially Blends With Glenohumeral Joint Capsule)

Innervation:
Posterior Axillary Nerve (C5-C6)

Blood Supply:
Posterior Humeral Circumflex Artery & Circumflex Scapular Artery

Function:
Brachium External Rotation; Humeral Head Stabilization

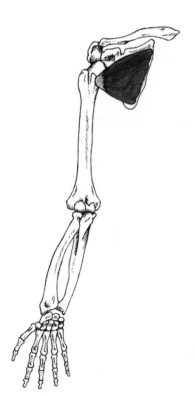

Subscapularis

Origin:
Subscapular Fossa

Insertion:
Lesser Tubercle Of Humerus (Partially Blends With Glenohumeral Joint Capsule)

Innervation:
Upper Subscapular Nerve & Lower Subscapular Nerve (C5-C6)

Blood Supply:
Suprascapular Artery, Axillary Artery, Subscapular Artery

Function:
Brachium Internal Rotation; Humeral Head Stabilization

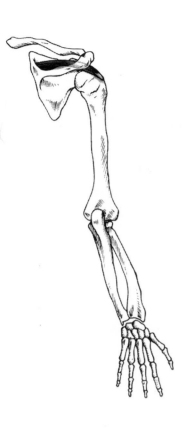

Supraspinatus

Origin:
Supraspinous Fossa Of Scapula

Insertion:
Superior Aspect, Greater Tuberosity
Of Humerus

Innervation:
Suprascapular Nerve (C5-C6)

Blood Supply:
Suprascapular Artery &
Dorsal Scapular Artery

Function:
Humerus Abduction, External Rotation

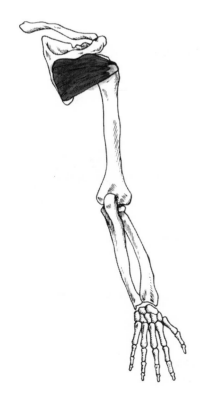

Infraspinatus

Origin:
Infraspinous Fossa Of Scapula

Insertion:
Dorsal Aspect, Middle Of Greater
Tuberosity Of Humerus

Innervation:
Suprascapular Nerve (C5-C6)

Blood Supply:
Suprascapular Artery &
Circumflex Scapular Artery

Function:
Brachium External Rotation;
Humeral Head Stabilization

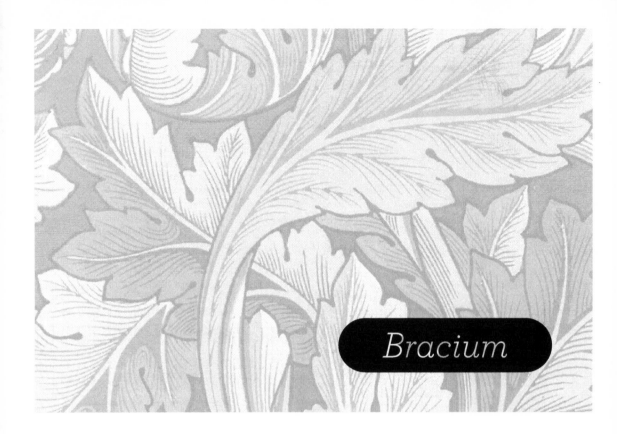

Bracium

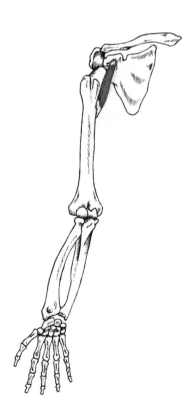

Coracobrachialis

Origin:
Coracoid Process Of Scapula

Insertion:
Medial Aspect Of Diaphysis
Of Humerus

Innervation:
Musculocutaneous Nerve (C5-C7)

Blood Supply:
Brachial Artery

Function:
Brachium Adduction, Flexion

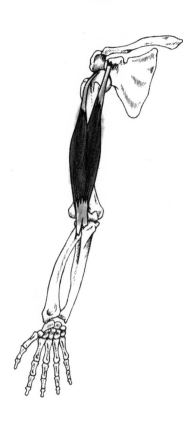

Biceps Brachii

Origin:
 Long Head– Supraglenoid Tubercle,
 Short Head– Coracoid Process

Insertion:
 Tuberosity Of Radius & Bicipital
 Aponeurosis To Proximal Ulna

Innervation:
 Musculocutaneous Nerve (C5-C6)

Blood Supply:
 Brachial Artery

Function:
 *Antebrachium Flexion; Shoulder Flexion; Brachium
 Adduction; Antebrachium Supination*

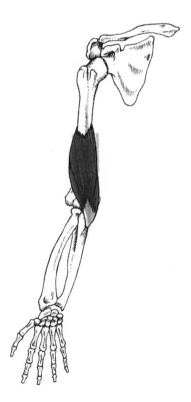

Brachialis

Origin:
 Ventral Aspect, Distal Humerus

Insertion:
 Tuberosity Of Ulna

Innervation:
 Musculocutaneous Nerve (C5-C7)

Blood Supply:
 Recurrent Radial Artery

Function:
 Antebrachium Flexion

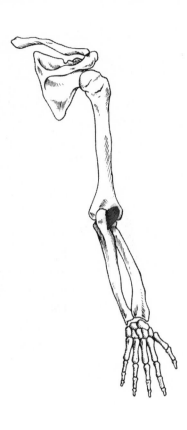

Anconeus

Origin:
Lateral Epicondyle Of Humerus

Insertion:
Lateral Olecranon

Innervation:
Radial Nerve (C6-C8)

Blood Supply:
Deep Brachial Artery, Recurrent
Interosseous Artery

Function:
*Assists With Antebrachium Extension; Elbow Joint
Stabilization During Pronation/Supination*

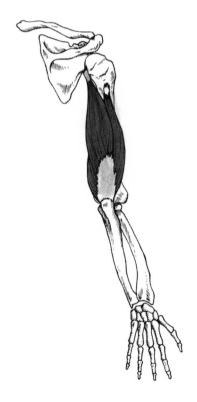

Triceps Brachii

Origin:
Lateral Head– Superior, Lateral Margin
Of Humerus; *Long Head–* Infraglenoid
Tubercle; *Medial Head–* Dorsal Aspect Of
Humerus (Distal To The Radial Groove)

Insertion:
Olecranon Of Ulna

Innervation:
Radial Nerve (C6-C8)

Blood Supply:
Deep Brachial Artery

Function:
Antebrachium Extension

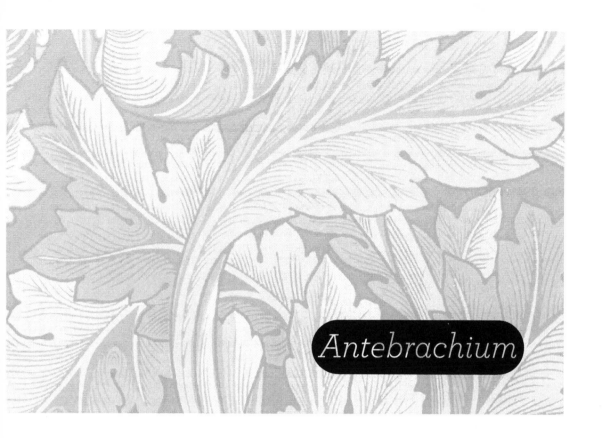

Antebrachium

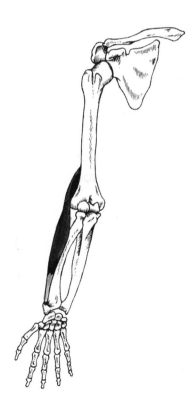

Brachioradialis

Origin:
Common Extensor Tendon: Lateral Epicondyle Of Humerus

Insertion:
Styloid Process Of Radius

Innervation:
Radial Nerve (C5-C6)

Blood Supply:
Radial Recurrent Artery

Function:
Elbow Flexion; Antebrachium Supination

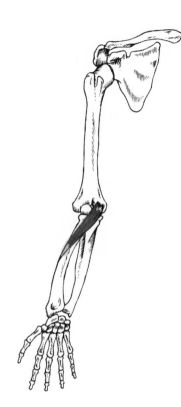

Pronator Teres

Origin:
Common Flexor Tendon: Medial
Supracondylar Ridge Of Humerus

Insertion:
Lateral Body Of Radius

Innervation:
Median Nerve (C6-C7)

Blood Supply:
Ulnar Artery; Radial Artery

Function:
Antebrachium Pronation

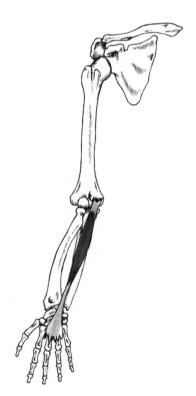

Palmaris Longus

Origin:
Common Flexor Tendon: Medial
Epicondyle Of Humerus

Insertion:
Palmar Aponeurosis

Innervation:
Median Nerve (C7-T1)

Blood Supply:
Ulnar Artery

Function:
Wrist Flexion

Flexor Carpi Radialis

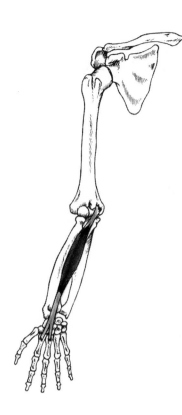

Origin:
Common Flexor Tendon: Medial Epicondyle Of Humerus

Insertion:
Palmar Aspect, Base Of Second & Third Metacarpals

Innervation:
Median Nerve (C6-C8)

Blood Supply:
Radial Artery

Function:
Wrist Flexion, Abduction

Flexor Carpi Ulnaris

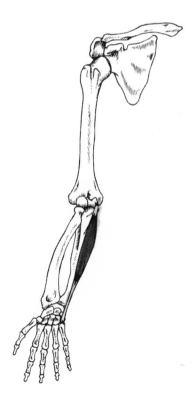

Origin:
Common Flexor Tendon: Medial Epicondyle Of Humerus

Insertion:
Palmar Aspect, Base Of Fifth Metacarpal & Pisiform

Innervation:
Ulnar Nerve (C7-C8)

Blood Supply:
Ulnar Artery

Function:
Wrist Flexion, Adduction

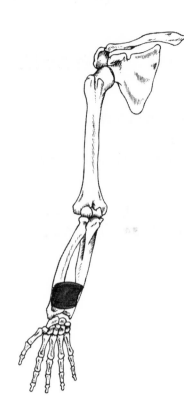

Pronator Quadratus

Origin:
Ventromedial Aspect Of Distal Ulna

Insertion:
Distal Ventrolateral Aspect Of Radius

Innervation:
Median Nerve (C7-T1)

Blood Supply:
Anterior Interosseous Artery

Function:
Antebrachium Pronation

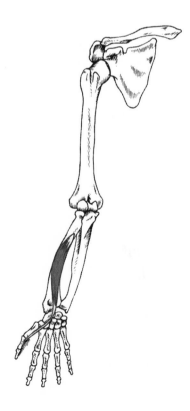

Flexor Pollicis Longus

Origin:
Ventral Aspect Of Radius &
Interosseous Membrane

Insertion:
Palmar Aspect, Base Of Distal Phalanx
Of Digit 1

Innervation:
Median Nerve (C7-T1)

Blood Supply:
Anterior Interosseous Artery

Function:
Thumb Flexion

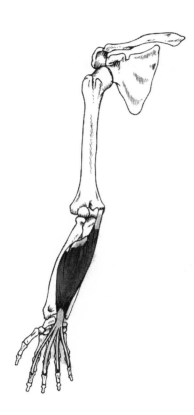

Flexor Digitorum Supeficialis

Origin:
Common Flexor Tendon: Medial
Epicondyle Of Humerus;
Ventral Aspect, Proximal Radius & Ulna

Insertion:
Palmar Aspect, Inserts As Two Slips To
Base Of Middle Phalanges Of Digits 2-5

Innervation:
Median Nerve (C7-T1)

Blood Supply:
Ulnar Artery

Function:
Finger Flexion At The Proximal
Interphalangeal Joints

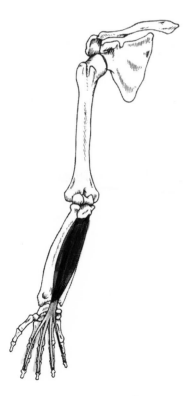

Flexor Digitorum Profundus

Origin:
Ventral Aspect Of Ulna; Anterior
Interosseous Membrane

Insertion:
Palmar Aspect, Base Of Distal Phalanges
Of Digits 2-5

Innervation:
Median Nerve (Radial Half, C8-T1);
Ulnar Nerve (Ulnar Half, C8-T1)

Blood Supply:
Anterior Interosseous Artery

Function:
Finger Flexion At The Proximal And Distal
Interphalangeal Joints

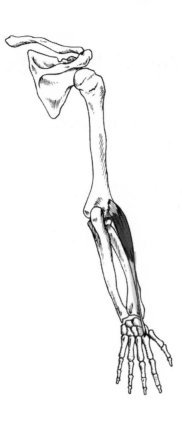

Extensor Carpi Radialis Longus

Origin:
Common Extensor Tendon: Lateral
Epicondyle Of Humerus

Insertion:
Dorsal Aspect, Base Of Second
Metacarpal

Innervation:
Radial Nerve (C6-C7)

Blood Supply:
Radial Artery

Function:
Wrist Extension, Abduction

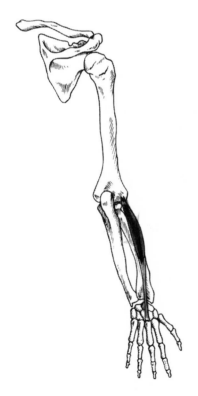

Extensor Carpi Radialis Brevis

Origin:
Common Extensor Tendon: Lateral
Epicondyle Of Humerus

Insertion:
Dorsal Aspect, Base Of Third Metacarpal

Innervation:
Radial Nerve- Deep Branch (C6-C7)

Blood Supply:
Radial Artery

Function:
Wrist Extension, Abduction

Extensor Carpi Ulnaris

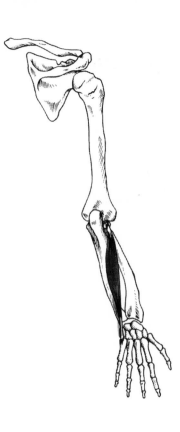

Origin:
Common Extensor Tendon: Lateral
Epicondyle Of Humerus

Insertion:
Dorsal Aspect, Base Of fifth Metacarpal

Innervation:
Radial Nerve– Deep Branch (C6-C8)

Blood Supply:
Ulnar Artery

Function:
Wrist Extension, Adduction

Supinator

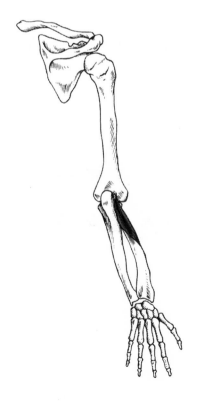

Origin:
Lateral Epicondyle Of Humerus &
Superior Crest Of Ulna

Insertion:
Lateral, Proximal Radial Shaft

Innervation:
Radial Nerve–Deep Branch (C5-C6)

Blood Supply:
Radial Recurrent Artery

Function:
Antebrachium Supination

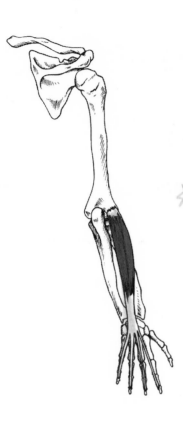

Extensor Digitorum

Origin:
Common Extensor Tendon: Lateral
Epicondyle Of Humerus

Insertion:
Extensor Expansion Of Middle & Distal
Phalanges Of Digits 2-5

Innervation:
Radial Nerve– Posterior Interosseous
Branch (C6-C8)

Blood Supply:
Posterior Interosseous Artery

Function:
Finger 2-5 Extension

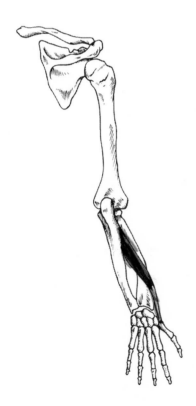

Abductor Pollicis Longus

Origin:
Dorsal Aspect Of Proximal Ulna, Radius
& Interosseous Membrane

Insertion:
Lateral Aspect, Base Of First Metacarpal

Innervation:
Radial Nerve– Posterior Interosseous
Branch (C6-C8)

Blood Supply:
Posterior Interosseous Artery

Function:
Thumb Abduction, Extension

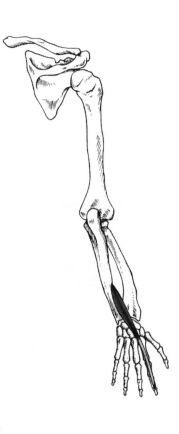

Extensor Indicis

Origin:
Dorsal Aspect, Distal Ulna &
Interosseous Membrane

Insertion:
Extensor Hood Of Digit 2

Innervation:
Radial Nerve– Posterior Interosseous
Branch (C6-C8)

Blood Supply:
Posterior Interosseous Artery

Function:
Index Finger Extension

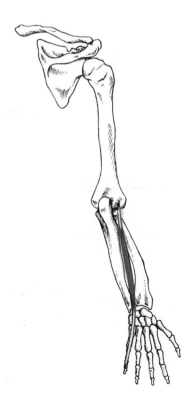

Extensor Digiti Minimi

Origin:
Common Extensor Tendon: Lateral
Epicondyle Of Humerus

Insertion:
Extensor Expansion At Proximal
Phalange Of Digit 5.

Innervation:
Radial Nerve– Posterior Interosseous
Branch (C6-C8)

Blood Supply:
Posterior Interosseous Artery

Function:
Pinky Finger Extension

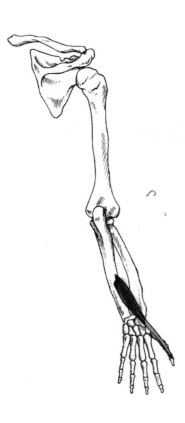

Extensor Pollicis Longus

Origin:
Dorsal Aspect Of Radius &
Interosseous Membrane

Insertion:
Dorsal Aspect, Base Of Distal Phalanx
Of Digit 1

Innervation:
Radial Nerve- Posterior Interosseous
Branch (C6-C8)

Blood Supply:
Posterior Interosseous Artery

Function:
Thumb Extension At Metacarpophalangeal Joint

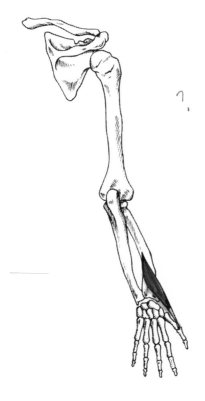

Extensor Pollicis Brevis

Origin:
Dorsal Aspect, Mid-Ulna &
Interosseous Membrane

Insertion:
Dorsal Aspect, Base Of Proximal
Phalanx Of Digit 1

Innervation:
Radial Nerve- Posterior Interosseous
Branch (C6-C8)

Blood Supply:
Posterior Interosseous Artery

Function:
Thumb Extension

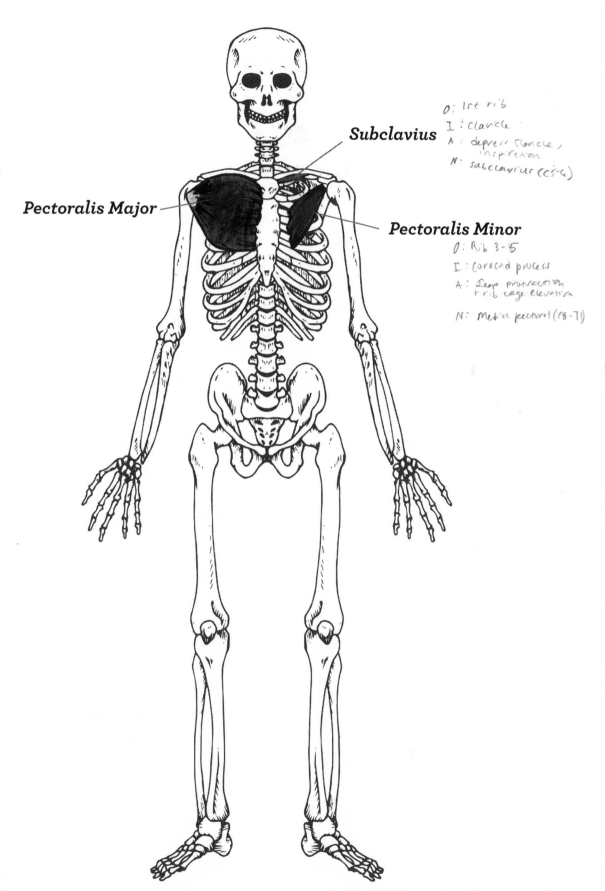

Subclavius

O: 1st rib

I: clavicle

A: depress clavicle, inspiration

N: subclavius (C5-6)

Pectoralis Major

Pectoralis Minor

O: Rib 3-5

I: Coracoid process

A: Scap protraction, rib cage elevation

N: Medial pectoral (C8-T1)

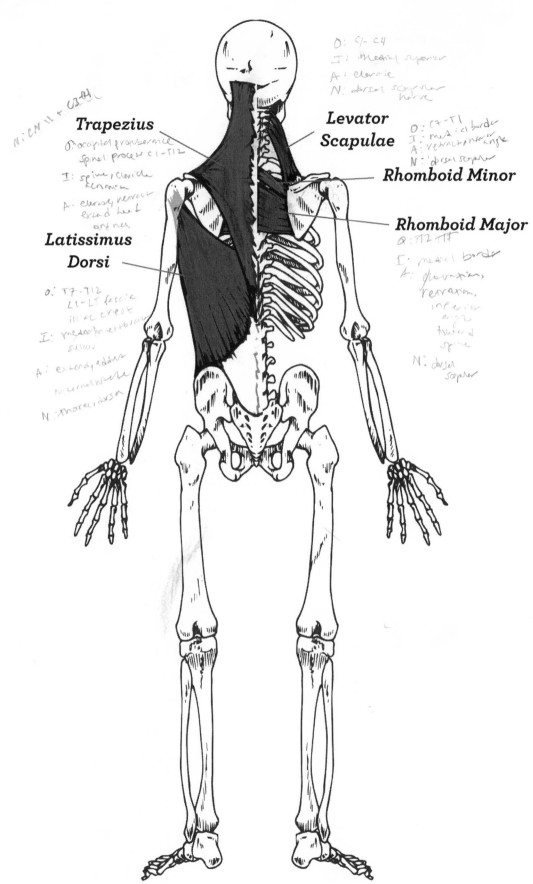

Trapezius

O: occipital protuberance
Spinal process C1-T12

I: spine, clavicle
acromion

A: elevate, retract
extend head
and neck

N: CN 11 + C3-C4

Latissimus Dorsi

O: T7-T12
L1-L5 fascia
iliac crest

I: medial intertubercular
sulcus

A: extend, adduct
internal rotate

N: thoracodorsal

Levator Scapulae

O: C1-C4
I: medial superior
A: elevate
N: dorsal scapular
nerve

Rhomboid Minor

O: C7-T1
I: medial border
A: retract anterior angle
N: dorsal scapular

Rhomboid Major

O: T12-T5
I: medial border
A: elevation,
retraction,
inferior
angle
toward
spine
N: dorsal
scapular

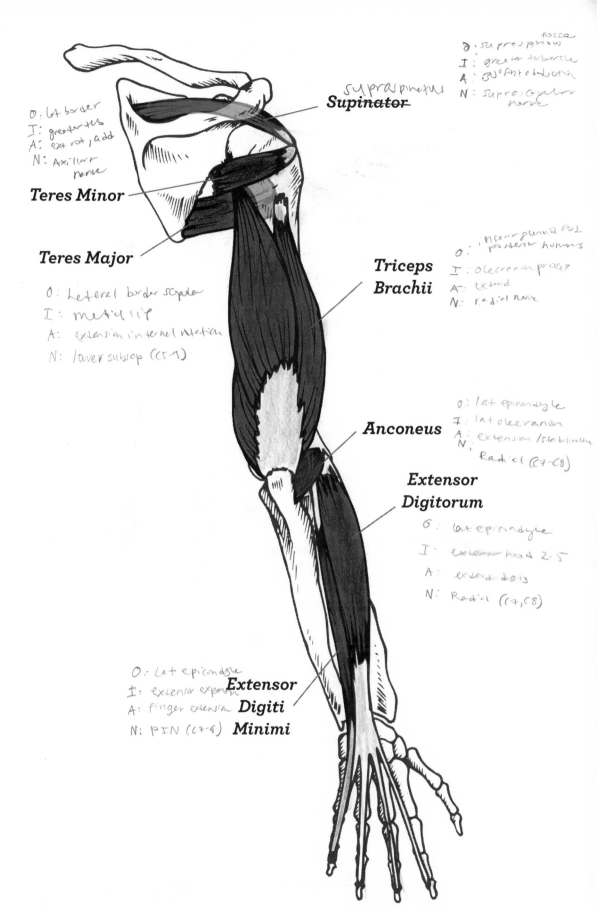

Supinator

supraspinatus

Teres Minor

O: lat border
I: greater tub
A: ext rot, add
N: Axillary nerve

Teres Major

O: Lateral border scapula
I: medial lip
A: extension internal rotation
N: lower subscap (C5-7)

Triceps Brachii

O: infraglenoid tub posterior humerus
I: Olecranon process
A: extend
N: radial nerve

Anconeus

O: lat epicondyle
I: lat olecranon
A: extension / stabilization
N: Radial (C7-C8)

Extensor Digitorum

O: lat epicondyle
I: extensor hood 2-5
A: extend digits
N: Radial (C7, C8)

O: Lat epicondyle
I: extensor expansion
A: finger extension
N: PIN (C7-8)

Extensor Digiti Minimi

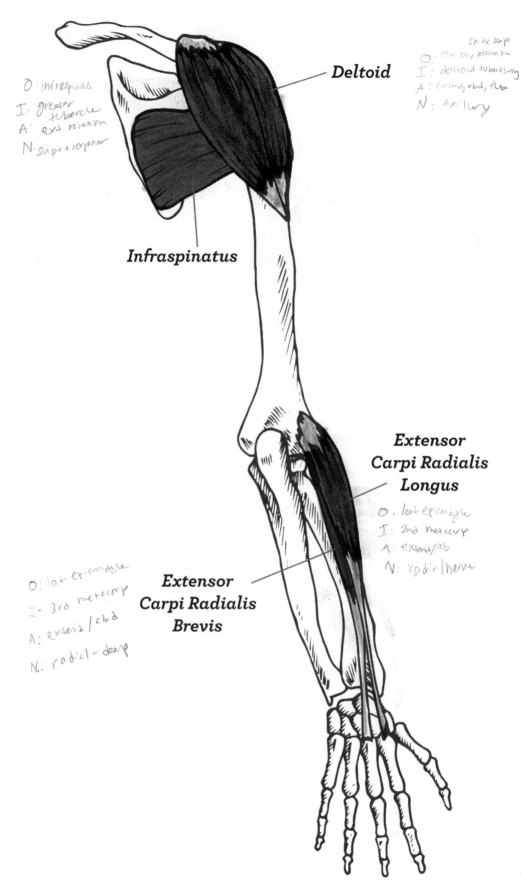

Deltoid

O: infraspinous

I: greater
tubercle

A: ext rotation

N: suprascapular

Spine scap
O: clavicle, acromion
I: deltoid tuberosity
A: extend, abd, flex
N: Axillary

Infraspinatus

**Extensor
Carpi Radialis
Longus**

O: lat epicondyle
I: 2nd metacarp
A: extend/abd
N: radial nerve

O: lat epicondyle
I: 3rd metacarp
A: extend/abd
N: radial - deep

**Extensor
Carpi Radialis
Brevis**

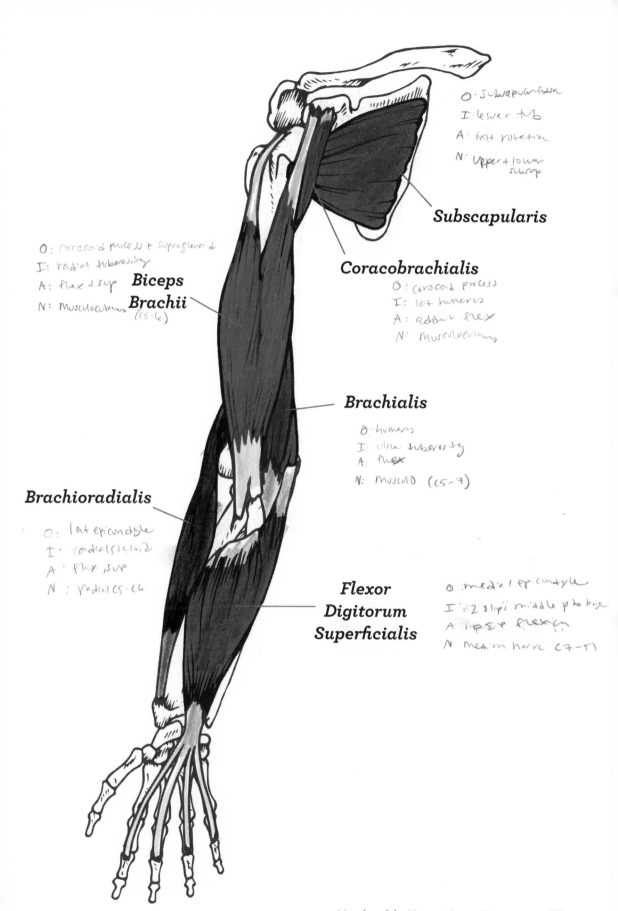

O: Subscapular fossa
I: lesser tub
A: int rotation
N: Upper + lower subscap

Subscapularis

O: coracoid process + supraglenoid
I: radial tuberosity
A: flex + sup
N: Musculocutaneus

Biceps Brachii (C5-6)

Coracobrachialis

O: coracoid process
I: lat humerus
A: adduct flex
N: Musculocutaneus

Brachialis

O: humerus
I: ulna tuberosity
A: flex
N: musculo (C5-7)

Brachioradialis

O: lat epicondyle
I: radial styloid
A: flex sup
N: radial C5-C6

Flexor Digitorum Superficialis

O: medial epicondyle
I: d2 slips middle phalanx
A: MP IP flexion
N: median nerve C7-T1

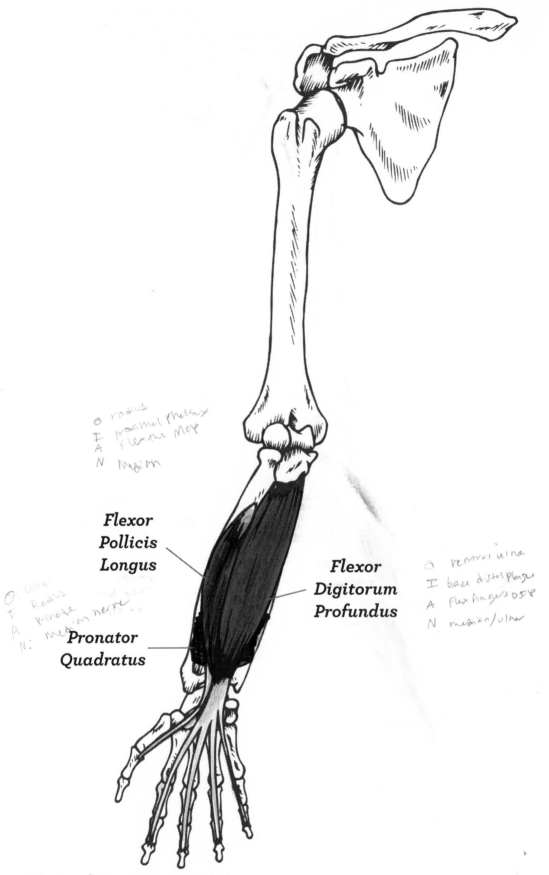

O radius
I proximal phalanx
A flex thu MCP
N Median

Flexor Pollicis Longus

O: ulna
I: Radius
A: Pronate
N: median nerve

Pronator Quadratus

Flexor Digitorum Profundus

O ventral ulna
I base distal phalanx
A Flex fingers DIP
N median/ulnar

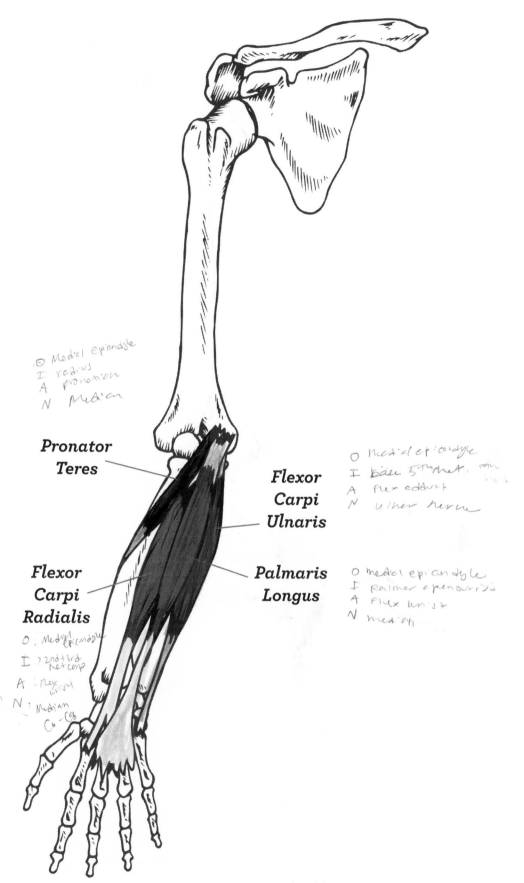

O Medial epicondyle
I radius
A pronation
N Median

Pronator Teres

Flexor Carpi Ulnaris

O Medial epicondyle
I base 5th met. on
A flex adduct
N ulnar nerve

Flexor Carpi Radialis

O: Medial epicondyle
I ? 2nd + 3rd met comp
A: Flex wrist
N: Median
C6 - C6

Palmaris Longus

O medial epicondyle
I palmar aponeurosis
A flex wrist
N median

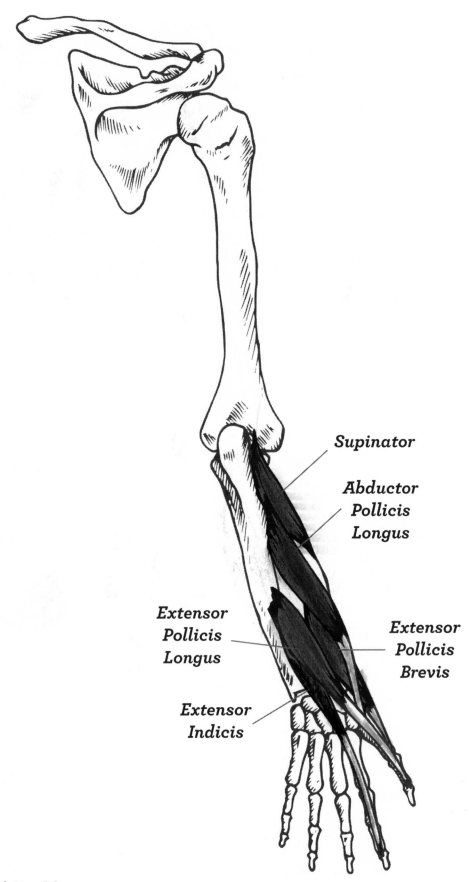

Supinator

Abductor
Pollicis
Longus

Extensor
Pollicis
Longus

Extensor
Pollicis
Brevis

Extensor
Indicis

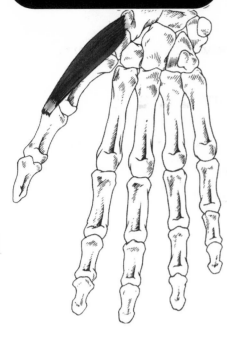

Abductor Pollicis Brevis

Origin:
Transverse Carpal Ligament, Scaphoid & Trapezium

Insertion:
Radial Base Of Proximal Phalanx Of Digit 1

Innervation:
Median Nerve- Recurrent Branch (C7-T1)

Blood Supply:
Superficial Palmar Arch

Function:
Thumb Abduction

Intrinsic

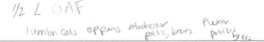

½ L OAF
lumbricals oppens abductor pollis brevis flexor pollicis brevis

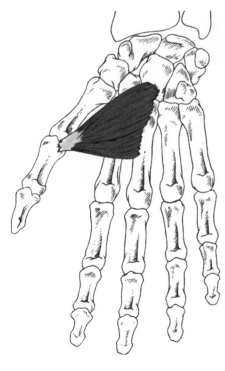

Adductor Pollicis

Origin:
Transverse Head- Anterior Body Of Third Metacarpal; Oblique Head- Base Of Second And Third Metacarpal, Trapezoid, & Capitate

Insertion:
Medial Side, Proximal Phalanx Of Digit 1

Innervation:
Ulnar Nerve- Deep Branch (C8-T1)

Blood Supply:
Deep Palmar Arch

Function:
Thumb Adduction; Aids In Opposition

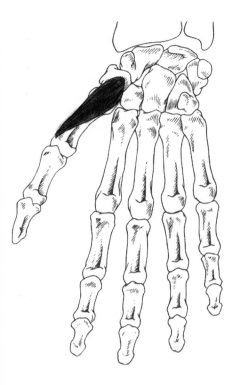

Opponens Pollicis

Origin:
  Trapezium & Transverse Carpal Ligament

Insertion:
  Radial Side Of First Metacarpal

Innervation:
  Median Nerve– Recurrent Branch (C7-T1)

Blood Supply:
  Superficial Palmar Arch

Function:
  Thumb Opposition

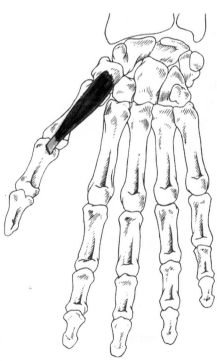

Flexor Pollicis Brevis

Origin:
  Trapezium & Flexor Retinaculum

Insertion:
  Proximal Phalanx Of Digit 1

Innervation:
  Median Nerve– Recurrent Branch (C7-T1)

Blood Supply:
  Superficial Palmar Arch   + deep branch
                             ulnar nerve
                             — medial head

Function:
  Thumb Flexion   MCP

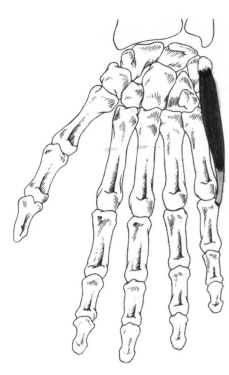

Abductor Digiti Minimi

Origin:
Pisiform & Flexor Retinaculum

Insertion:
Anterior, Base Of Proximal Phalanx Of Digit 5

Innervation:
Ulnar Nerve– Deep Branch (C8-T1)

Blood Supply:
Ulnar Artery

Function:
Pinky Finger Abduction

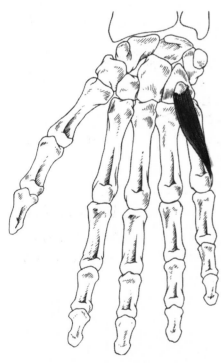

Opponens Digiti Minimi

Origin:
Hook Of Hamate & Flexor Retinaculum

Insertion:
Medial Border Of 5Th Metacarpal

Innervation:
Ulnar Nerve– Deep Branch (C8-T1)

Blood Supply:
Ulnar Artery

Function:
Pinky Finger Opposition

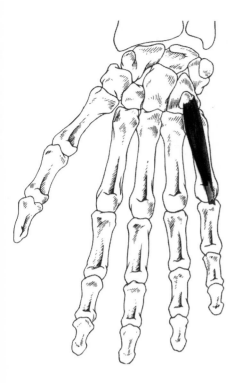

Flexor Digiti Minimi

Origin:
 Hook Of Hamate

Insertion:
 Ventral Aspect, Base Of Proximal Phalanx Of Digit 5

Innervation:
 Ulnar Nerve- Deep Branch (C8-T1)

Blood Supply:
 Ulnar Artery

Function:
 Pinky Finger Flexion

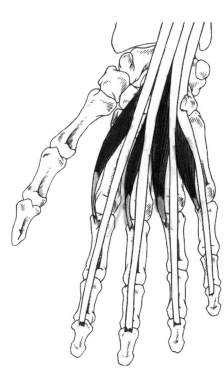

Lumbricals

Origin:
Tendons Of Flexor Digitorum Profundus

Insertion:
Extensor Expansion Of Digits 2-5

Innervation:
1st & 2nd Lumbricals Median Nerve;
3rd & 4th Lumbricals Ulnar Nerve-
Deep Branch (C7-T1)

Blood Supply:
Superficial Palmar Arch, Deep Palmar Arch

Function:
Finger Flexion At Metacarpophalangeal Joint And
Extension At Interphalangeal Joints

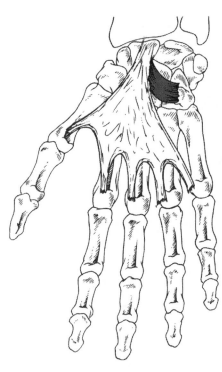

Palmaris Brevis

Origin:
Flexor Retinaculum, &
Palmar Aponeurosis

Insertion:
Skin Of Palm

Innervation:
Ulnar Nerve- Superficial Branch (C7-T1)

Blood Supply:
Palmar Metacarpal Artery

Function:
Pulls On Skin Over Hypothenar Eminence

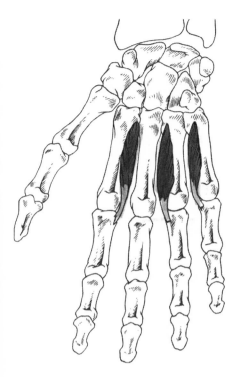

Palmar Interossei

Origin:
    Medial Aspect Of Metacarpals 2, 4, 5

Insertion:
    Bases Of Proximal Phalanges Of
    Corresponding Digit

Innervation:
    Ulnar Nerve- Deep Branch (C8-T1)

Blood Supply:
    Palmar Metacarpal Artery Of
    Deep Palmar Arch

Function:
    Finger Adduction

PAD

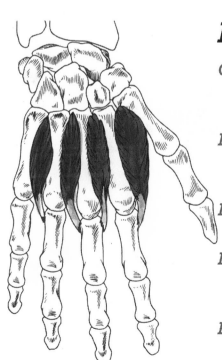

Dorsal Interossei

Origin:
    Each Interossei Is Attached To Both
    The Metacarpals It Is Between

Insertion:
    Proximal Phalanges, Extensor
    Expansions Of Digits 2-4

Innervation:
    Ulnar Nerve- Deep Branch (C8-T1)

Blood Supply:
    Dorsal Metacarpal Artery, Palmar
    Metacarpal Artery

Function:
    Finger Abduction

DAB

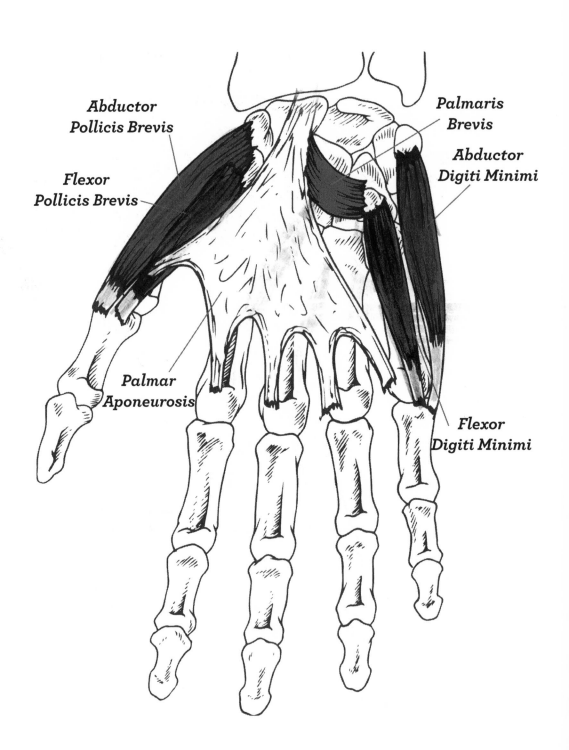

Abductor
Pollicis Brevis

Flexor
Pollicis Brevis

Palmaris
Brevis

Abductor
Digiti Minimi

Palmar
Aponeurosis

Flexor
Digiti Minimi

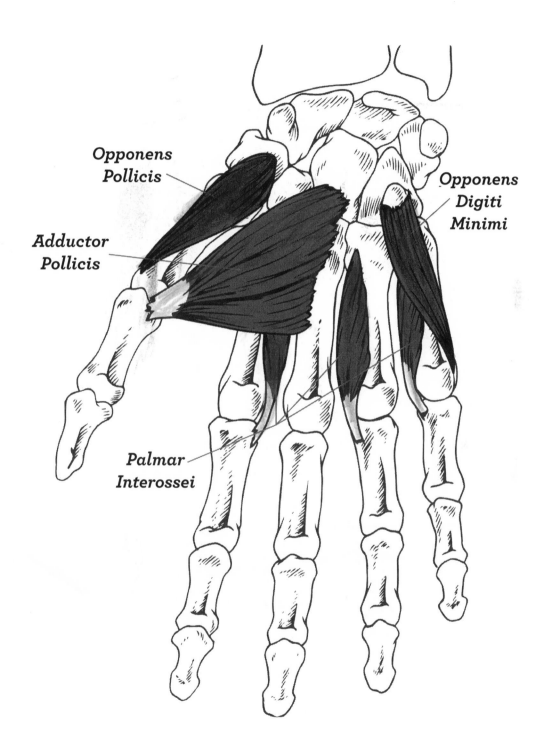

Opponens
Pollicis

Adductor
Pollicis

Opponens
Digiti
Minimi

Palmar
Interossei

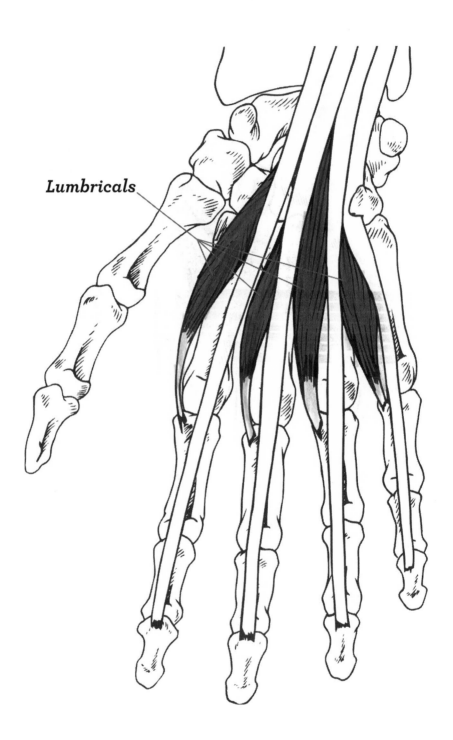

Lumbricals

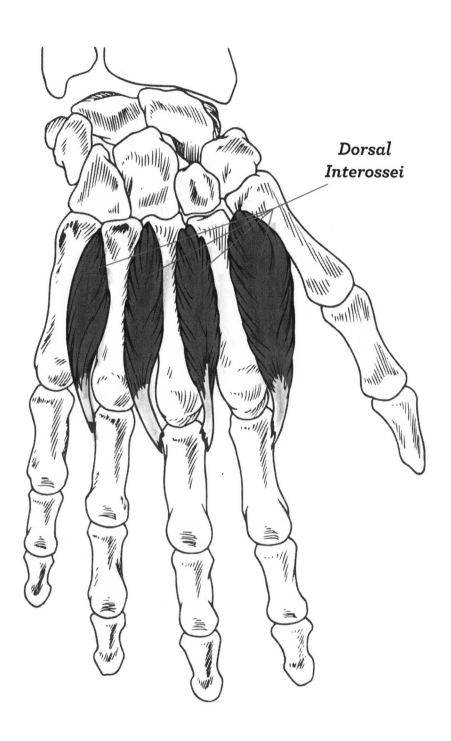

Dorsal Interossei

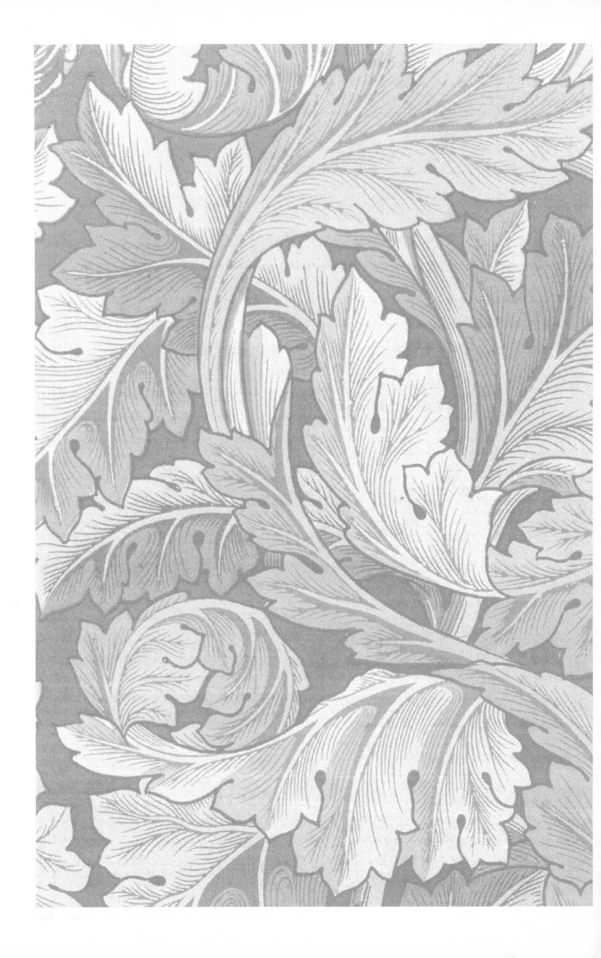

LOWER EXTREMITY

Lumbar Plexus

Like the Brachial Plexus, the Lumbar Plexus gives rise to a number of large nerves that supplies muscles of the lower extremity, low abdomen and pelvic bowl.

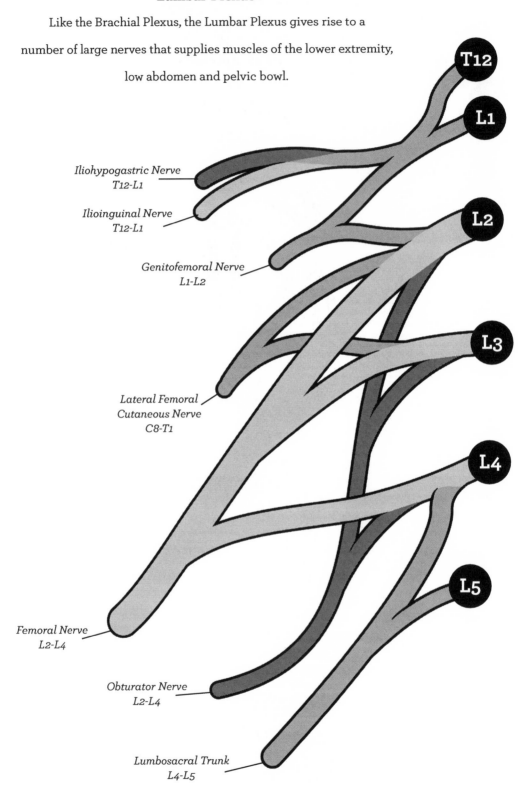

Iliohypogastric Nerve
T12-L1

Ilioinguinal Nerve
T12-L1

Genitofemoral Nerve
L1-L2

Lateral Femoral
Cutaneous Nerve
C8-T1

Femoral Nerve
L2-L4

Obturator Nerve
L2-L4

Lumbosacral Trunk
L4-L5

T12

L1

L2

L3

L4

L5

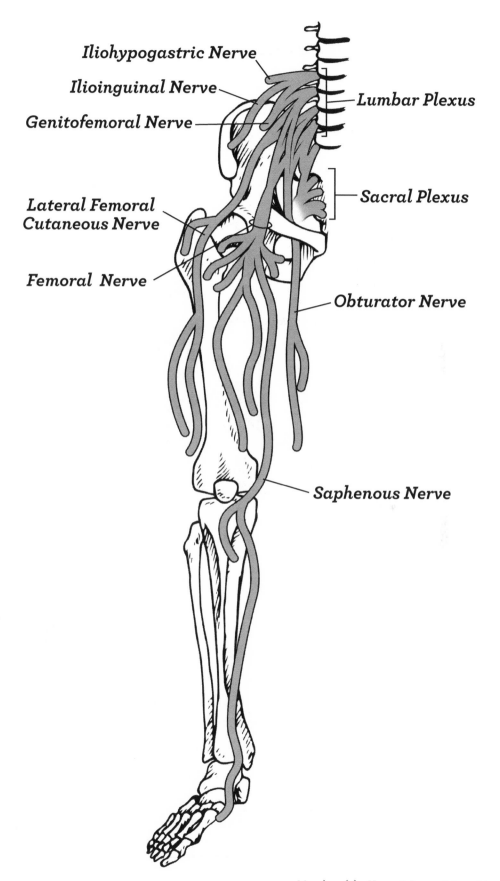

Iliohypogastric Nerve

Ilioinguinal Nerve

Genitofemoral Nerve

Lumbar Plexus

Sacral Plexus

Lateral Femoral
Cutaneous Nerve

Femoral Nerve

Obturator Nerve

Saphenous Nerve

Sacral Plexus

The Sacral Plexus works in harmony with the Lumbar plexus to innervate the lower extremity. While the Lumbar Plexus supplies mainly the ventromedial thigh, the sacral plexus controls the dorsolateral portion.

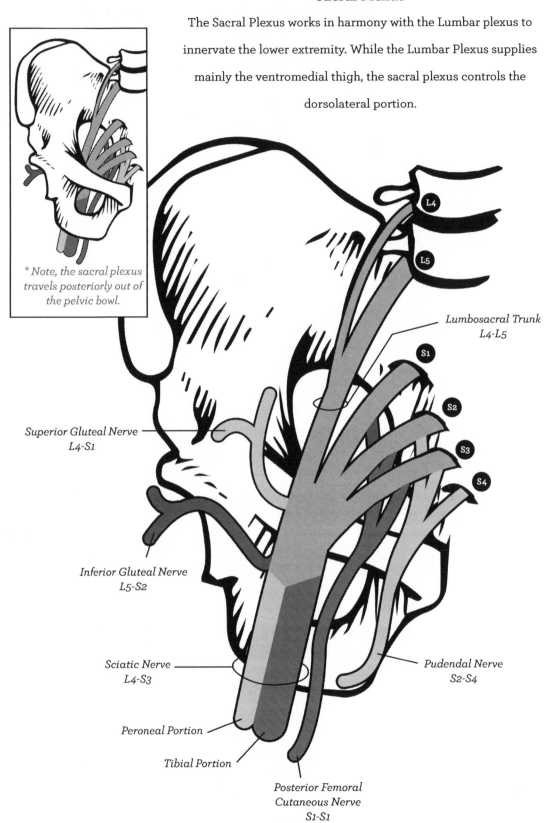

Note, the sacral plexus travels posteriorly out of the pelvic bowl.

L4

L5

S1

S2

S3

S4

Lumbosacral Trunk
L4-L5

Superior Gluteal Nerve
L4-S1

Inferior Gluteal Nerve
L5-S2

Sciatic Nerve
L4-S3

Pudendal Nerve
S2-S4

Peroneal Portion

Tibial Portion

Posterior Femoral
Cutaneous Nerve
S1-S1

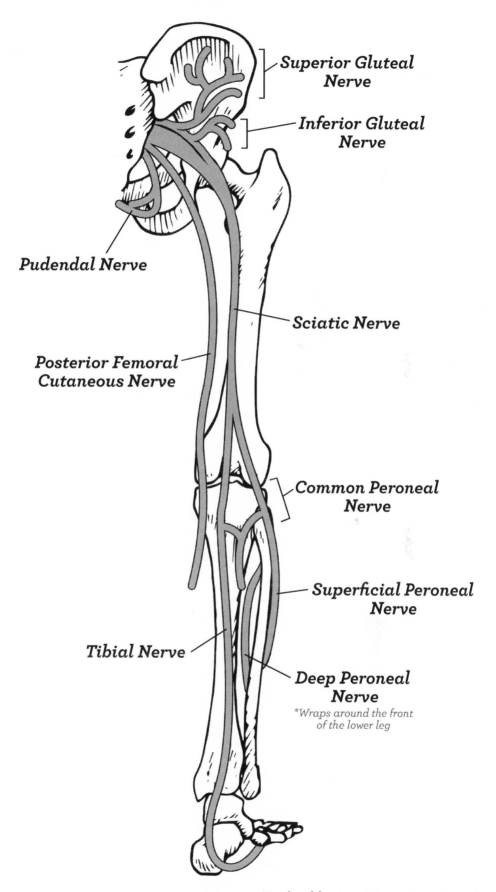

Superior Gluteal
Nerve

Inferior Gluteal
Nerve

Pudendal Nerve

Sciatic Nerve

Posterior Femoral
Cutaneous Nerve

Common Peroneal
Nerve

Superficial Peroneal
Nerve

Tibial Nerve

Deep Peroneal
Nerve
*Wraps around the front
of the lower leg

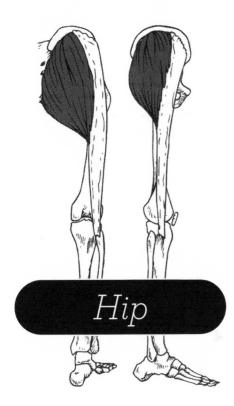

Gluteus Maximus

Origin:
Superolateral Ilium, Lateral Sacrum, & Sacrotuberous Ligament

Insertion:
Gluteal Tuberosity & Iliotibial Tract

Innervation:
Inferior Gluteal Nerve (L5-S2)

Blood Supply:
Superior And Inferior Gluteal Arteries

Function:
Femur Extension, External Rotation

Hip

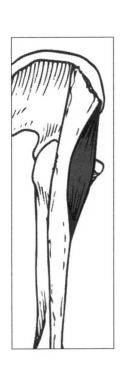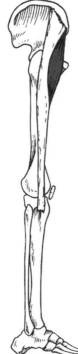

Tensor Fasciae Latae

Origin:
Iliac Crest, Within The IT Band

Insertion:
Gerdy's Tubercle Via The IT Band

Innervation:
Superior Gluteal Nerve (L4-S1)

Blood Supply:
Lateral Circumflex Femoral Artery, Superior Gluteal Artery

Function:
Hip Flexion, Medial Rotation

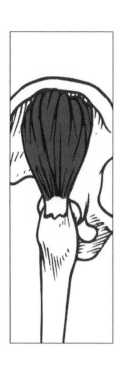

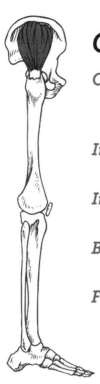

Gluteus Medius

Origin:
Gluteal Surface Of Ilium, Located
Underneath Gluteus Maximus

Insertion:
Greater Trochanter Of Femur

Innervation:
Superior Gluteal Nerve (L4-S1)

Blood Supply:
Superior Gluteal Artery

Function:
Hip Abduction (Works With Gluteus Minimus)

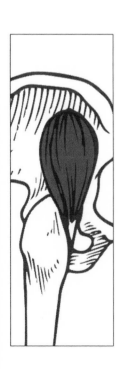

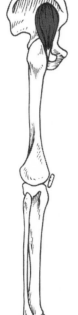

Gluteus Minimus

Origin:
Gluteal Surface Of Ilium, Located
Underneath Gluteus Medius

Insertion:
Greater Trochanter Of Femur

Innervation:
Superior Gluteal Nerve (L4-S1)

Blood Supply:
Superior Gluteal Artery

Function:
Hip Abduction (Works With Gluteus Medius)

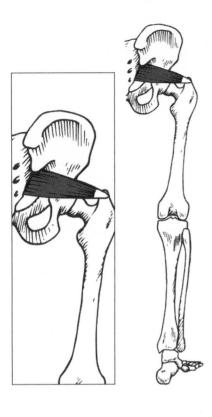

Piriformis

Origin:
Ventrolateral Aspect Sacrum

Insertion:
Greater Trochanter

Innervation:
Nerve To Piriformis (S1-S2)

Blood Supply:
Inferior Gluteal, Lateral Sacral &
Superior Gluteal Artery

Function:
Hip External Rotation

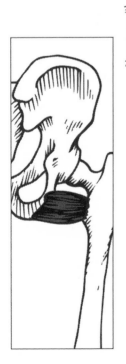
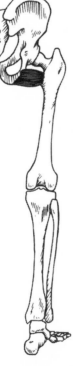

Quadratus Femoris

Origin:
Ischial Tuberosity

Insertion:
Intertrochanteric Crest Of Femur

Innervation:
Nerve To Quadratus Femoris (L4-S1)

Blood Supply:
Medial Circumflex Artery

Function:
Hip Lateral Rotation; Thigh Adduction

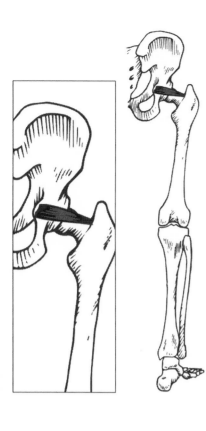

Superior Gemellus

Origin:
Spine Of Ischium

Insertion:
Greater Trochanter Of Femur, Medial Aspect

Innervation:
Nerve To Obturator Internus (S1-S2)

Blood Supply:
Inferior Gluteal Artery

Function:
Hip Lateral Rotation

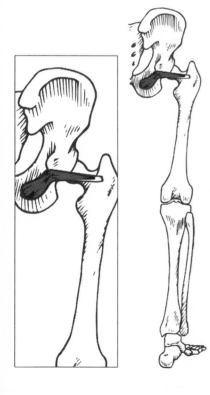

Obturator Internus

Origin:
Dorsal Aspect Of Obturator Membrane

Insertion:
Greater Trochanter Of Femur, Medial Aspect

Innervation:
Nerve To Obturator Internus (S1-S2)

Blood Supply:
Inferior Gluteal Artery

Function:
Hip Lateral Rotation

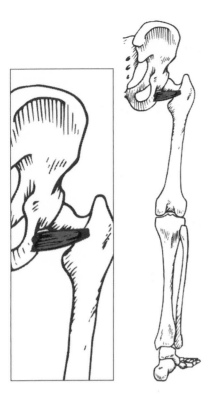

Inferior Gemellus

Origin:
  Ischial Tuberosity

Insertion:
  Greater Trochanter Of Femur, Medial Aspect

Innervation:
  Nerve To Quadratus Femoris (S1-S2)

Blood Supply:
  Inferior Gluteal Artery

Function:
  Hip Lateral Rotation

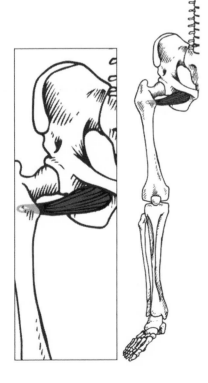

Obturator Externus

Origin:
  Obturator Foramen & Obturator Membrane

Insertion:
  Trochanteric Fossa Of Femur

Innervation:
  Obturator Nerve- Posterior Branch (L3-L4)

Blood Supply:
  Obturator Artery

Function:
  Hip Lateral Rotation; Thigh Adduction

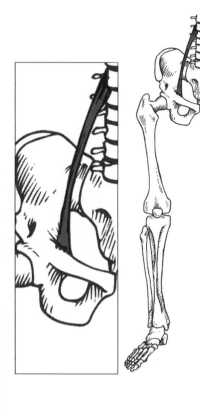

Psoas Minor

Origin:
Lateral Aspect Of T12 And L1 Vertebral
Bodies & Disc

Insertion:
Pectineal Line/Iliopubic Eminence

Innervation:
Ventral Ramus (L1)

Blood Supply:
Lumbar Branch Of Iliolumbar Artery

Function:
Contributes To Trunk Flexion

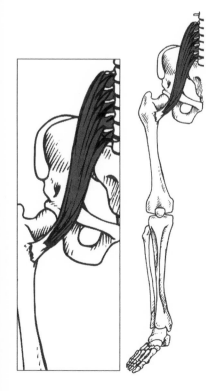

Psoas Major

Origin:
T12-L5 Transverse Processes & Lateral
Aspect Of Discs Between The Vertebra

Insertion:
Lesser Trochanter Of Femur

Innervation:
Ventral Rami (L2-L4)

Blood Supply:
Lumbar Branch Of Iliolumbar Artery

Function:
Femur/Trunk Flexion

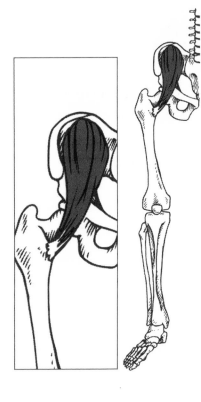

Iliacus

Origin:
Iliac Fossa, Superior Two Thirds

Insertion:
Lesser Trochanter Of Femur

Innervation:
Femoral Nerve (L2-L4)

Blood Supply:
Iliac Branch Of Iliolumbar Artery And
Medial Femoral Circumflex Artery

Function:
Femur/Trunk Flexion

Thigh

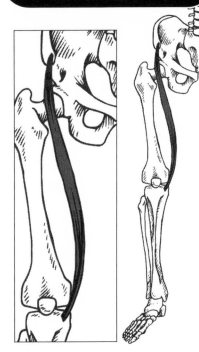

Sartorius

Origin:
ASIS (Anterior Superior Iliac Spine)

Insertion:
Pes Anserinus– Anteriomedial Aspect
Of Proximal Tibia

Innervation:
Femoral Nerve (L2-L4)

Blood Supply:
Femoral Artery

Function:
Hip Flexion, Abduction, Lateral Rotation;
Knee Flexion

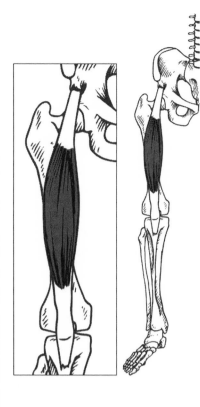

Rectus Femoris

Origin:
AIIS (Anterior Inferior Iliac Spine)
& Acetabulum

Insertion:
Quadriceps Tendon/Patellar Tendon

Innervation:
Femoral Nerve (L2-L4)

Blood Supply:
Lateral Femoral Circumflex Artery

Function:
Knee Extension; Hip Flexion

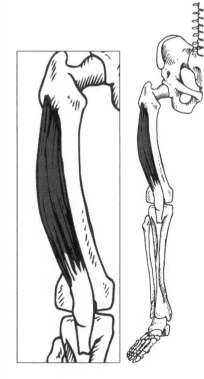

Vastus Lateralis

Origin:
Lateral Linea Aspera, Intertrochanteric
Line, Base Of Greater Trochanter

Insertion:
Quadriceps Tendon/Patellar Tendon

Innervation:
Femoral Nerve (L2-L4)

Blood Supply:
Lateral Femoral Circumflex Artery

Function:
Knee Extension

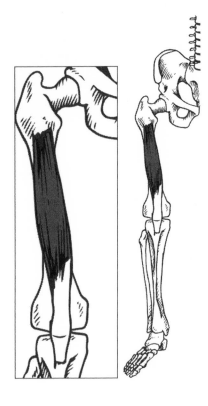

Vastus Intermedius

Origin:
Anterolateral Shaft Of Femur, Directly Underneath Rectus Femoris

Insertion:
Quadriceps Tendon/Patellar Tendon

Innervation:
Femoral Nerve (L2-L4)

Blood Supply:
Femoral Artery

Function:
Knee Extension

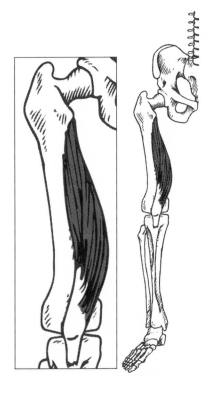

Vastus Medialis

Origin:
Medial Aspect Of Femur

Insertion:
Quadriceps Tendon/Patellar Tendon

Innervation:
Femoral Nerve (L2-L4)

Blood Supply:
Femoral Artery

Function:
Knee Extension

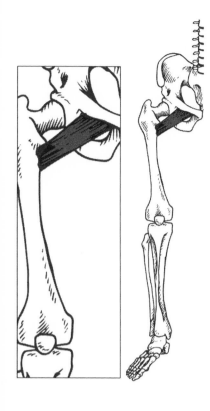

Pectineus

Origin:
Pectineal Line Of Pubic Bone

Insertion:
Pectineal Line Of Femur

Innervation:
Femoral Nerve And/Or Obturator
Nerve (L2-L4)

Blood Supply:
Obturator Artery

Function:
Thigh Adduction

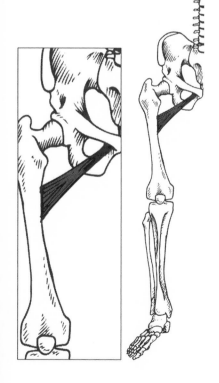

Adductor Brevis

Origin:
Ventral Aspect Of Inferior Ramus/
Body Of Pubic Bone

Insertion:
Lesser Trochanter/Linea Aspera

Innervation:
Obturator Nerve (L2-L4)

Blood Supply:
Deep Femoral Artery

Function:
Thigh Adduction

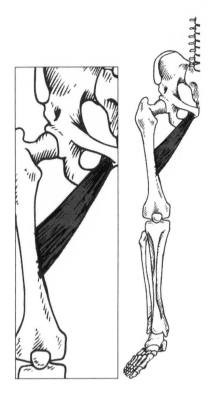

Adductor Longus

Origin:
Pubic Body, Inferior To The Pubic Crest

Insertion:
Middle Third Of Linea Aspera

Innervation:
Obturator Nerve– Anterior Branch (L2-L4)

Blood Supply:
Deep Femoral Artery

Function:
Thigh Adduction

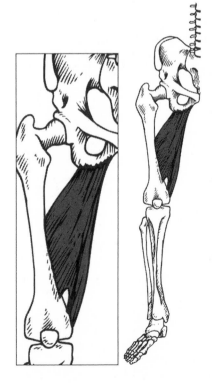

Adductor Magnus

Origin:
Pubic Bone & Ischial Tuberosity

Insertion:
Linea Aspera & Adductor Tubercle
Of Femur

Innervation:
Obturator Nerve– Posterior Branch (L2-S1)

Blood Supply:
Deep Femoral Artery

Function:
Thigh Adduction, Hip Extension

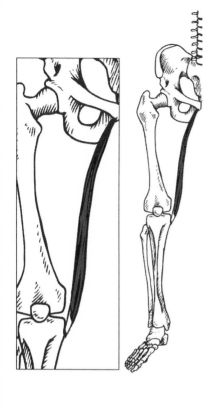

Gracilis

Origin:
Ischiopubic Ramus

Insertion:
Pes Anserinus– Anteriomedial Aspect
Of Proximal Tibia

Innervation:
Obturator Nerve– Anterior Branch
(L2-L4)

Blood Supply:
Medial Femoral Circumflex Artery

Function:
Hip Adduction

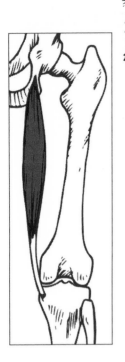
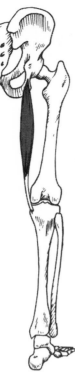

Semitendinosus

Origin:
Ischial Tuberosity

Insertion:
Pes Anserinus– Anteriomedial Aspect
Of Proximal Tibia

Innervation:
Sciatic Nerve– Tibial Portion (L5-S2)

Blood Supply:
Inferior Gluteal Arteries And
Perforating Arteries

Function:
Knee Flexion; Hip Extension

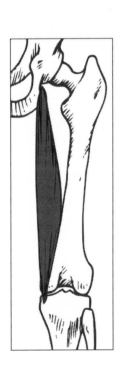
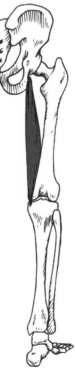

Semimembranosus

Origin:
Ischial Tuberosity

Insertion:
Medial Condyle Of Tibia

Innervation:
Sciatic Nerve– Tibial Portion (L5-S2)

Blood Supply:
Deep Femoral Artery And Gluteal Arteries

Function:
Knee Flexion; Hip Extension

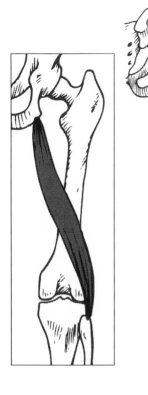

Biceps Femoris- Long Head

Origin:
Ischial Tuberosity

Insertion:
Head Of Fibula/Lateral Tibial Condyle

Innervation:
Sciatic Nerve- Tibial Portion (L5-S2)

Blood Supply:
Deep Femoral Artery

Function:
Knee Flexion; Hip Extension

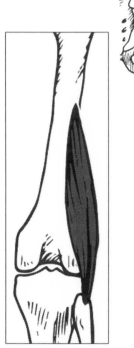
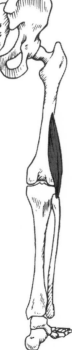

Biceps Femoris- Short Head

Origin:
Linea Aspera

Insertion:
Head Of Fibula/Lateral Tibial Condyle

Innervation:
Sciatic Nerve- Peroneal Portion (L5-S2)

Blood Supply:
Deep Femoral Artery

Function:
Knee Flexion; Hip Extension

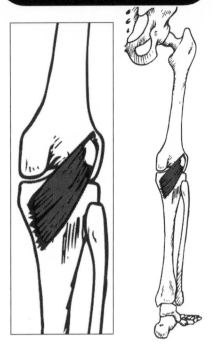

Popliteus

Origin:
Lateral Femoral Condyle

Insertion:
Posterior Tibia, Proximal End Of Diaphysis

Innervation:
Tibial Nerve (L4-S1)

Blood Supply:
Popliteal Artery

Function:
Femur Lateral Rotation (When Standing); Tibia Medial Rotation (When Femur Is Fixed); Assists In Knee Flexion

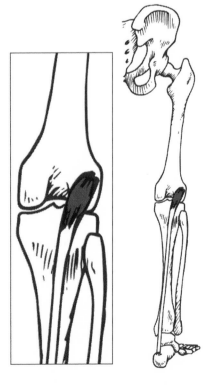

Plantaris

Origin:
Lateral Supracondylar Ridge Of Femur

Insertion:
Medial Calcaneus
(Underneath Gastrocnemius)

Innervation:
Tibial Nerve (S1-S2)

Blood Supply:
Sural Artery

Function:
Ankle Flexion; Foot Plantar Flexion

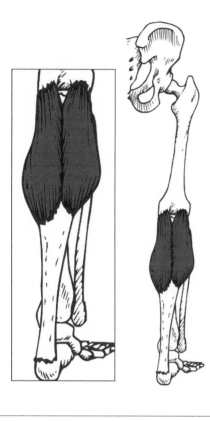

Gastrocnemius

Origin:
Lateral & Medial Femoral Condyles

Insertion:
Calcaneus (Via Achilles Tendon)

Innervation:
Tibial Nerve (L5-S2)

Blood Supply:
Sural Artery

Function:
Ankle Plantar Flexion; Knee Flexion

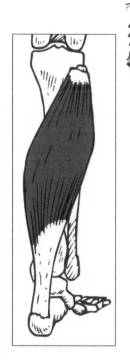
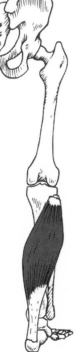

Soleus

Origin:
Soleal Line Of Tibia & Fibula

Insertion:
Calcaneus

Innervation:
Tibial Nerve (L5-S2)

Blood Supply:
Popliteal Artery, Posterior Tibial Artery, Peroneal Artery

Function:
Ankle Plantar Flexion

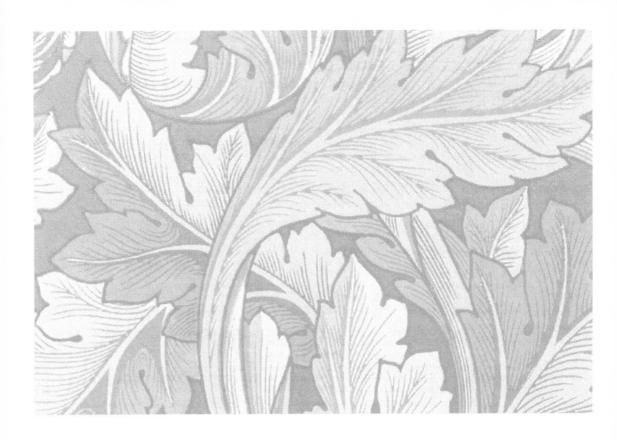

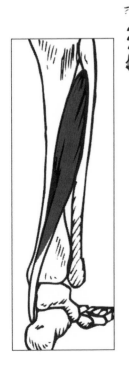
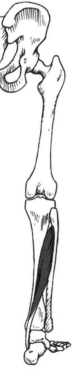

Tibialis Posterior

Origin:
Dorsal Aspect, Proximal Tibia, Fibula
& Interosseous Membrane

Insertion:
Navicular Bone

Innervation:
Tibial Nerve (L5-S1)

Blood Supply:
Posterior Tibial Artery

Function:
Foot Inversion; Ankle Plantar Flexion

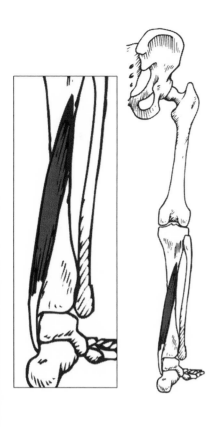

Flexor Digitorum Longus

Origin:
Dorsal Aspect, Middle Third Of Tibia

Insertion:
Plantar Aspect Of Distal Phalanges,
Digits 2-5

Innervation:
Tibial Nerve (L5-S1)

Blood Supply:
Posterior Tibial Artery

Function:
Lateral Four Digit Flexion

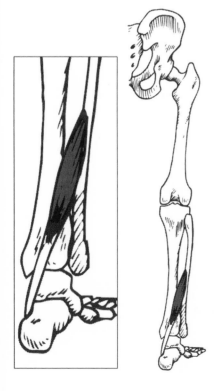

Flexor Hallucis Longus

Origin:
Dorsal Aspect, Middle Third Of Fibula
& Interosseous Membrane

Insertion:
Plantar Aspect Of Distal Phalanx
Of Digit 1

Innervation:
Tibial Nerve (L5-S2)

Blood Supply:
Peroneal Artery

Function:
Big Toe Flexion (All Joints); Ankle Plantar Flexion

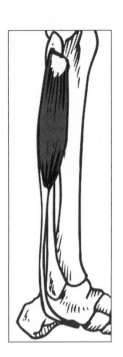
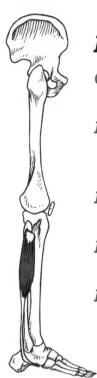

Peroneus Longus

Origin:
    Proximal, Lateral Shaft Of Fibula

Insertion:
    Plantar Aspect, Base Of First
    Metatarsal & Cuneiform

Innervation:
    Superficial Peroneal Nerve (L4-S1)

Blood Supply:
    Peroneal Artery

Function:
    Ankle Plantar Flexion; Foot Eversion

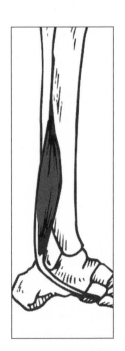
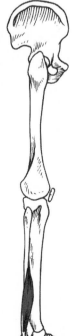

Peroneus Brevis

Origin:
    Distal Two-Thirds Of Lateral Shaft
    Of Fibula

Insertion:
    Base Of Fifth Metatarsal

Innervation:
    Superficial Peroneal Nerve (L4-S1)

Blood Supply:
    Peroneal Artery

Function:
    Ankle Plantar Flexion; Foot Eversion

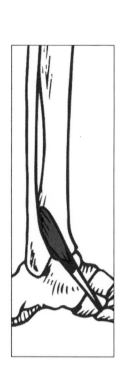

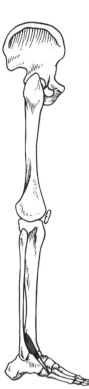

Peroneus Tertius

Origin:
Ventral Aspect, Distal Third Of Shaft
Of Fibula

Insertion:
Dorsal Surface Of Fifth Metatarsal

Innervation:
Deep Peroneal Nerve (L4-S1)

Blood Supply:
Anterior Tibial Artery

Function:
Ankle Dorsiflexion; Foot Eversion

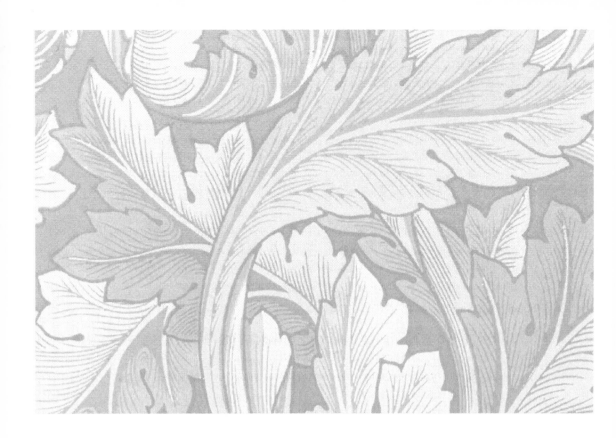

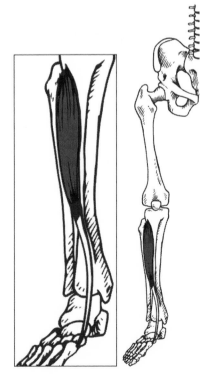

Tibialis Anterior

Origin:
Lateral Condyle & Upper Half Of
Anterior Tibia

Insertion:
Medial Cuneiform & First Metatarsal Bone

Innervation:
Deep Peroneal Nerve (L4-S1)

Blood Supply:
Anterior Tibial Artery

Function:
Ankle Dorsiflexion; Foot Inversion

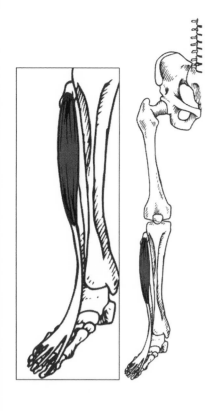

Extensor Digitorum Longus

Origin:
  Ventral Aspect, Lateral Condyle
  Of Tibia, Anterior Shaft Of Tibia
  & Proximal Three Quarters Of
  Interosseous Membrane

Insertion:
  Dorsal Aspect Of Middle & Distal
  Phalanges Of Digits 2-5

Innervation:
  Deep Peroneal Nerve (L4-S1)

Blood Supply:
  Anterior Tibial Artery

Function:
  Lateral Four Toe Extension; Ankle Dorsiflexion

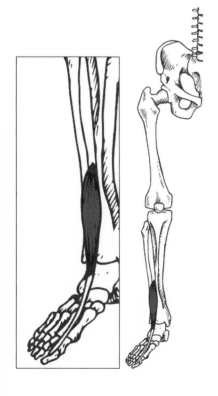

Extensor Hallucis Longus

Origin:
  Ventral Aspect, Middle Portion Of
  Fibula & Interosseous Membrane

Insertion:
  Dorsal Aspect Of Distal Phalanx
  Of Digit 1

Innervation:
  Deep Peroneal Artery (L5-S1)

Blood Supply:
  Anterior Tibial Artery

Function:
  Big Toe Extension; Assists In Ankle Dorsiflexion

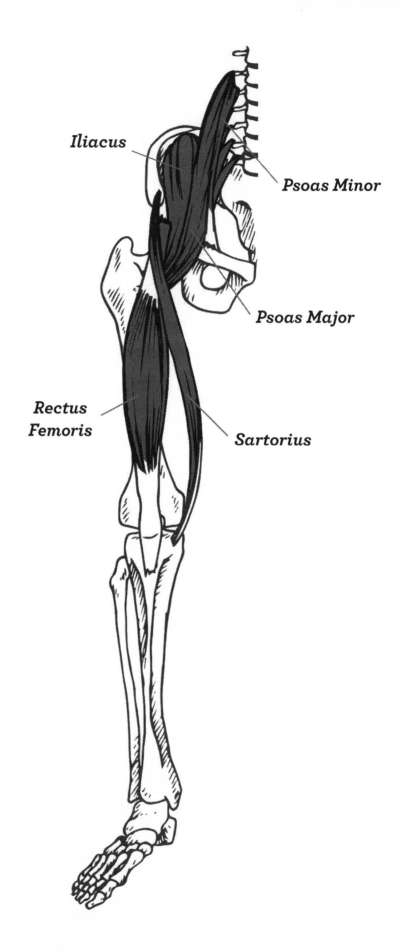

Iliacus

Psoas Minor

Psoas Major

Rectus
Femoris

Sartorius

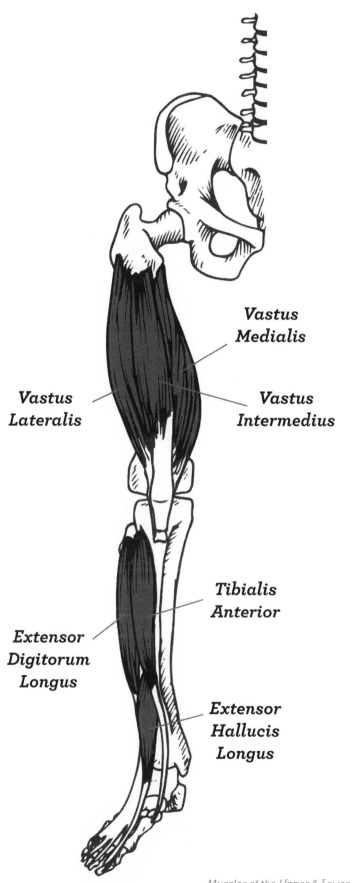

Vastus
Medialis

Vastus
Lateralis

Vastus
Intermedius

Tibialis
Anterior

Extensor
Digitorum
Longus

Extensor
Hallucis
Longus

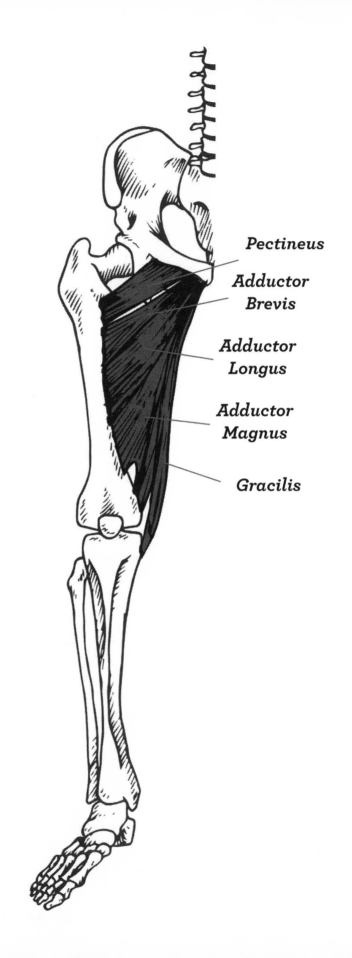

Pectineus

Adductor
Brevis

Adductor
Longus

Adductor
Magnus

Gracilis

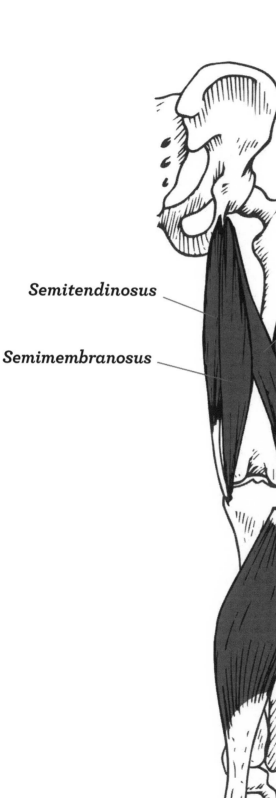

Semitendinosus

Semimembranosus

Long Head
Biceps Femoris

Short Head
Biceps Femoris

Soleus

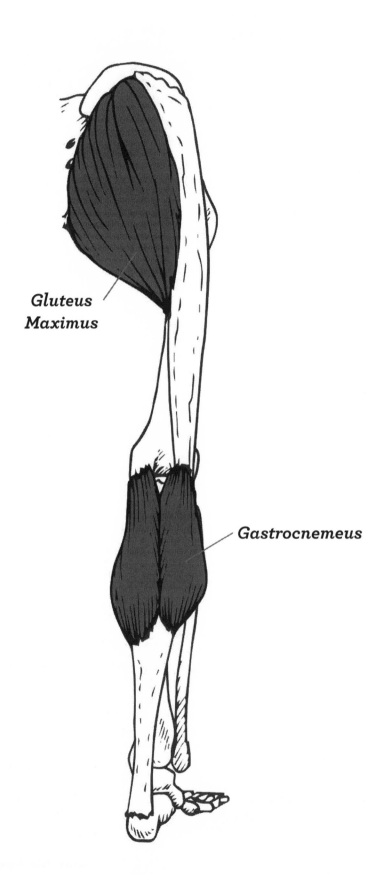

Gluteus
Maximus

Gastrocnemeus

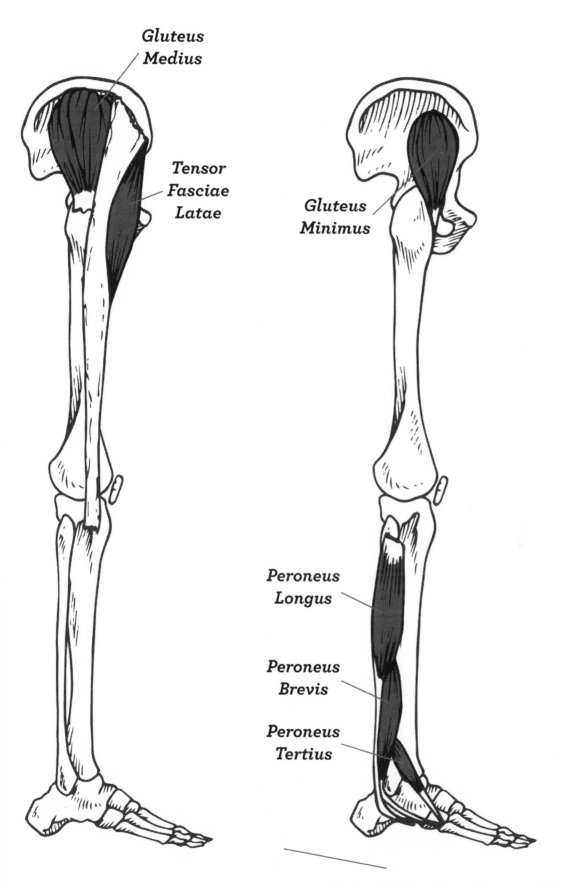

Gluteus
Medius

Tensor
Fasciae
Latae

Gluteus
Minimus

Peroneus
Longus

Peroneus
Brevis

Peroneus
Tertius

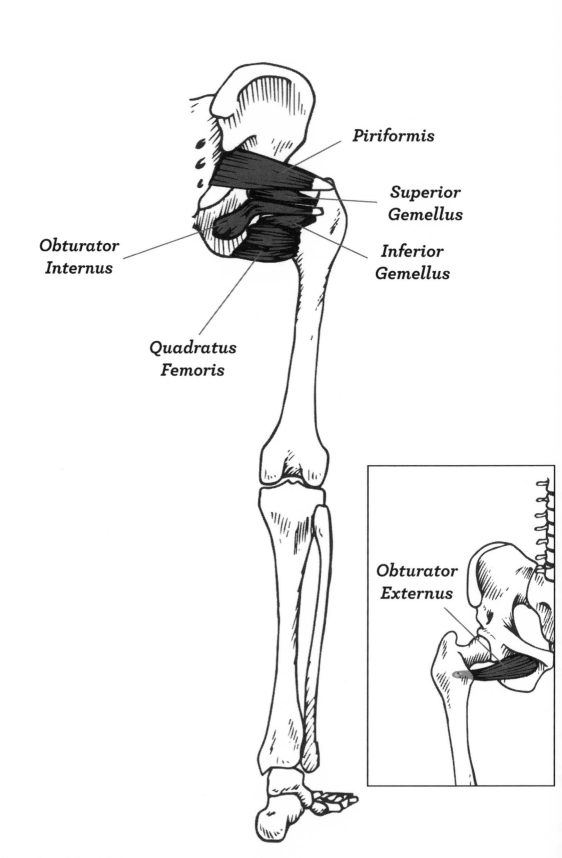

Piriformis

Superior
Gemellus

Inferior
Gemellus

Obturator
Internus

Quadratus
Femoris

Obturator
Externus

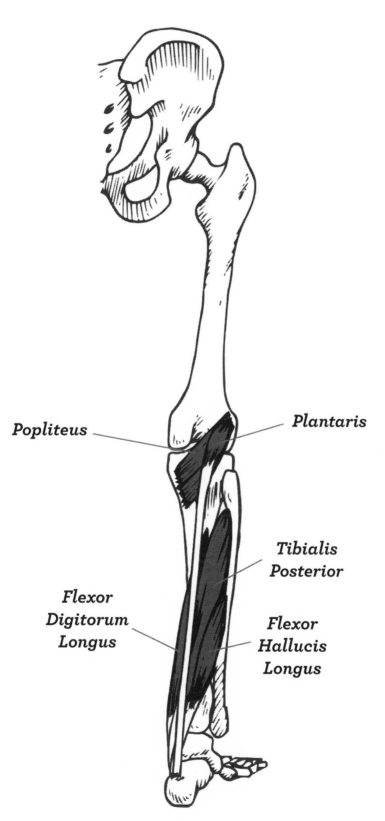

Popliteus

Plantaris

Tibialis Posterior

Flexor Digitorum Longus

Flexor Hallucis Longus

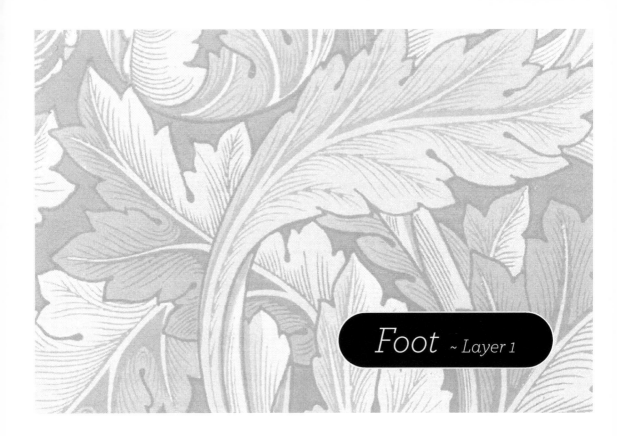

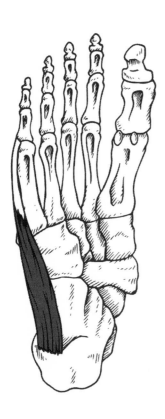

Abductor Digiti Minimi

Origin:
Plantar Aponeurosis & Calcaneus

Insertion:
Lateral Aspect, Base Of Proximal
Phalanx Of Digit 5

Innervation:
Lateral Plantar Nerve (S1-S2)

Blood Supply:
Lateral Plantar Artery

Function:
Big Toe Abduction, Supports Transverse Arch Of Foot

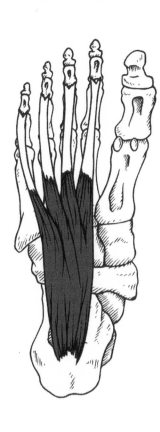

Flexor Digitorum Brevis

Origin:
Plantar Aponeurosis &
Calcaneal Tuberosity

Insertion:
Base Of Middle Phalanges Of Digits 2-5

Innervation:
Medial Plantar Nerve (S1-S2)

Blood Supply:
Medial And Lateral Plantar Arteries

Function:
Lateral Four Toe Flexion

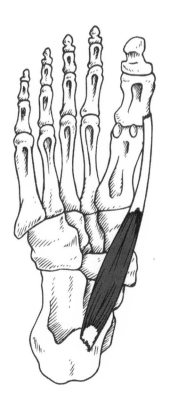

Abductor Hallucis

Origin:
Calcaneal Tuberosity

Insertion:
Medial Aspect Of Base Of Proximal
Phalanx Of Digit 1

Innervation:
Medial Plantar Nerve (S1-S2)

Blood Supply:
Medial Plantar Artery

Function:
Big Toe Abduction

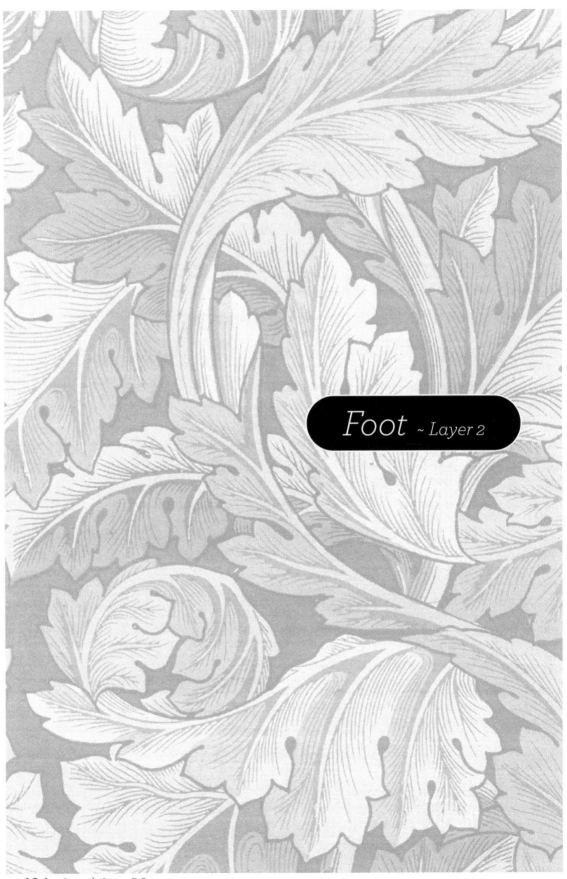

Foot ~ Layer 2

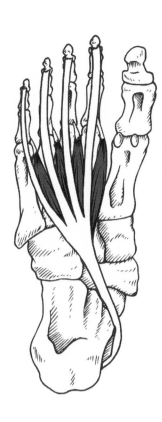

Lumbricals

Origin:
Flexor Digitorum Longus Tendon

Insertion:
Medial Aspect Of Base Of Proximal
Phalanges Of Digits 2-5

Innervation:
Medial & Lateral Plantar Nerves (L5-S2)

Blood Supply:
Lumbrical 1– Medial Plantar Artery;
Lumbicals 2-4– Lateral Plantar Artery

Function:
*Lateral 4 Toe Flexion At Metatarsophalangeal
Joint; Extension At Interphalageal Joint*

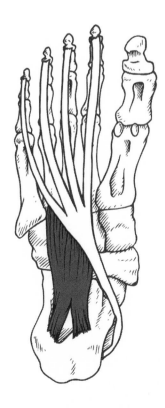

Quadratus Plantae

Origin:
Calcaneus

Insertion:
Tendon Of Flexor Digitorum Longus

Innervation:
Lateral Plantar Nerve (S1-S2)

Blood Supply:
Medial & Lateral Plantar Arteries

Function:
*Assists Flexor Digitorum Longus In Lateral
Four Toe Flexion*

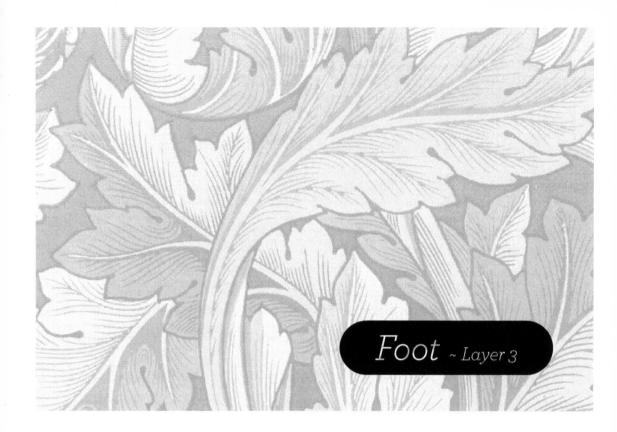

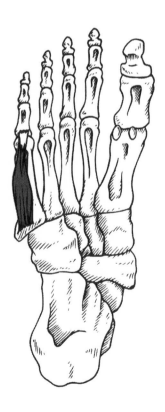

Flexor Digiti Minimi

Origin:
  Base Of Fifth Metatarsal

Insertion:
  Base Of Proximal Phalanx Of Digit 5

Innervation:
  Lateral Plantar Nerve-
  Superficial Branch (S1-S2)

Blood Supply:
  Lateral Plantar Artery

Function:
  Pinky Toe Flexion

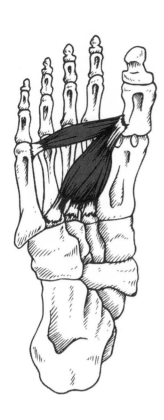

Adductor Hallucis

Origin:
    Oblique Head– Base Of Metatarsals
    2-4; Transverse Head– Metatarsophalangeal
    Joints Of Digits 3-5

Insertion:
    Lateral Aspect, Base Of Proximal
    Phalanx Of Digit 1

Innervation:
    Lateral Plantar Nerve (S1-S2)

Blood Supply:
    Lateral Plantar Artery

Function:
    Big Toe Adduction

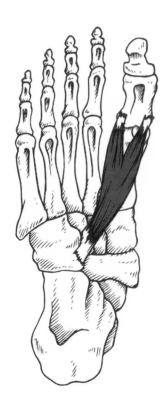

Flexor Hallucis Brevis

Origin:
    Plantar Aspect Of Cuboid & Lateral
    Cuneiform Bones

Insertion:
    Base Of Proximal Phalanx Of Digit 1

Innervation:
    Medial Plantar Nerve (S1-S2)

Blood Supply:
    Medial Plantar Artery

Function:
    Big Toe Flexion

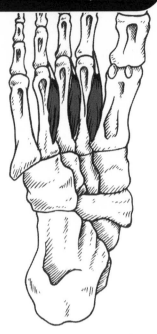

Plantar Interossei

Origin:
Medial Aspect, Bodies Of Third To Fifth Metatarsals

Insertion:
Medial Aspect, Base Of Proximal Phalanx Of Corresponding Digit

Innervation:
Tibial Nerve (L5-S2)

Blood Supply:
Lateral Plantar Nerve (S1-S2)

Blood Supply: Plantar Artery

Function:
Toes 3-5 Adduction

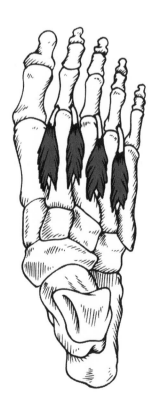

Dorsal Interossei

Origin:
Medial Aspect Of Both Metatarsals

Insertion:
Interossei 1– Medial Aspect, Base Of Proximal Phalanx Of Digit 2;
Interossei 2-4– Lateral Aspect, Base Of Proximal Phalanges Of Digits 2-4

Innervation:
Lateral Plantar Nerve (S1-S2)

Blood Supply:
Lateral Plantar Artery

Function:
Toes 2-4 Abduction

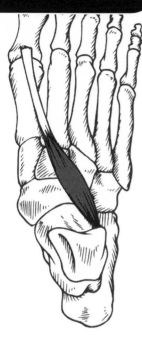

Extensor Hallucis Brevis

Origin:
Anterior, Superior Aspect Of Calcaneus

Insertion:
Dorsal Aspect Of Digit 1 Proximal Phalanx

Innervation:
Deep Peroneal Nerve (L5-S1)

Blood Supply:
Dorsal Pedal Artery

Function:
Big Toe Extension

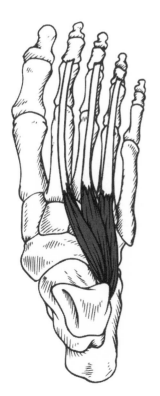

Extensor Digitorum Brevis

Origin:
Anterior, Superior Aspect Of Calcaneus

Insertion:
Dorsal Aspect, Base Of Middle Phalanges
Digits 2-4

Innervation:
Deep Peroneal Nerve (L5-S1)

Blood Supply:
Dorsal Pedal Artery

Function:
Toes 2-4 Extension

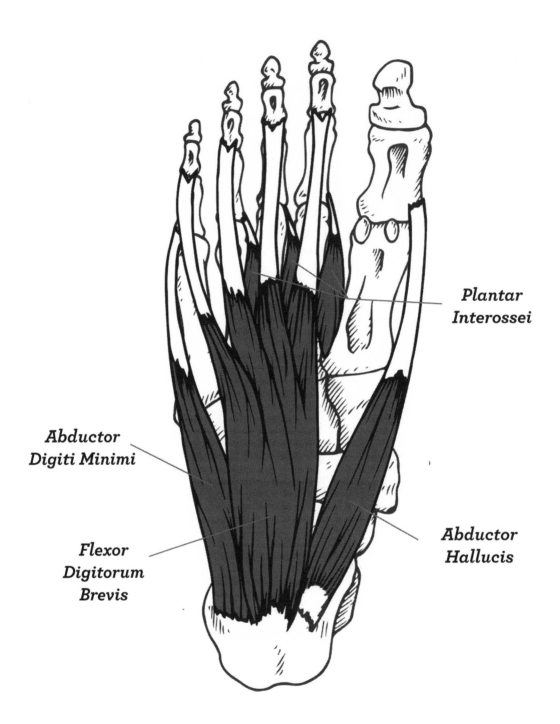

Plantar
Interossei

Abductor
Digiti Minimi

Flexor
Digitorum
Brevis

Abductor
Hallucis

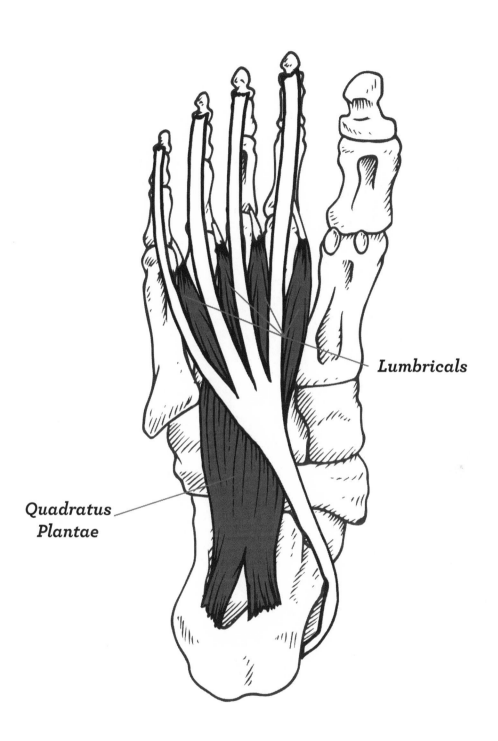

Lumbricals

Quadratus Plantae

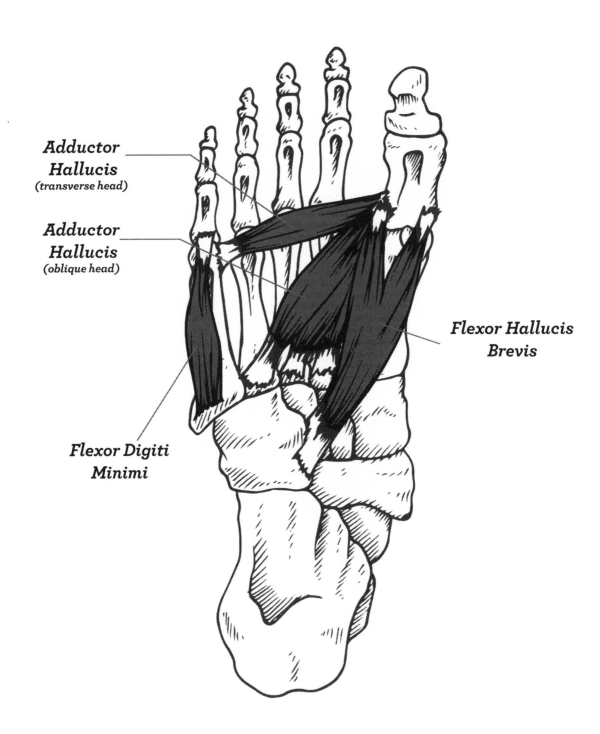

**Adductor
Hallucis**
(transverse head)

**Adductor
Hallucis**
(oblique head)

**Flexor Digiti
Minimi**

**Flexor Hallucis
Brevis**

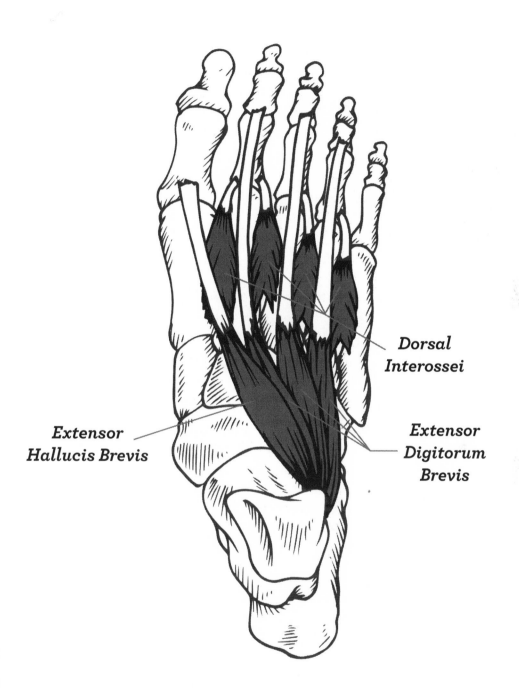

Dorsal Interossei

Extensor Hallucis Brevis

Extensor Digitorum Brevis

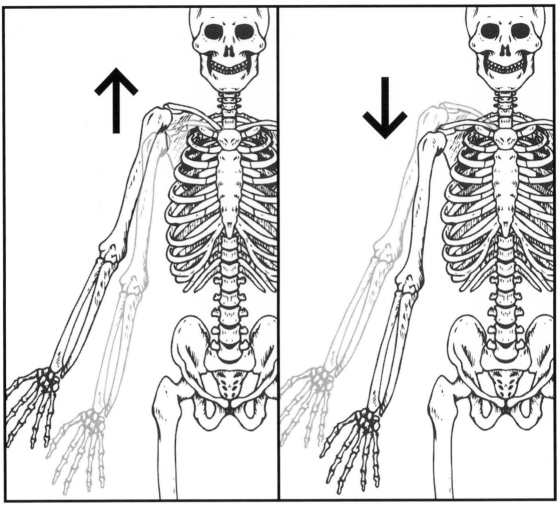

Shoulder: Elevation   *Shoulder: Depression*

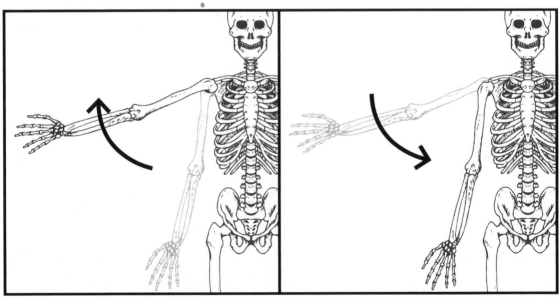

Arm: Abduction   *Arm: Adduction*

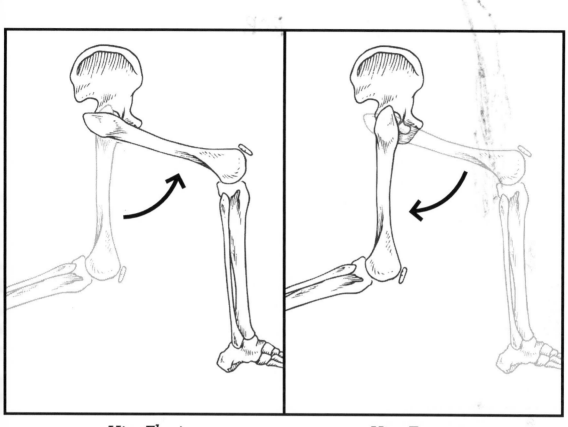

Hip: Flexion

Hip: Extension

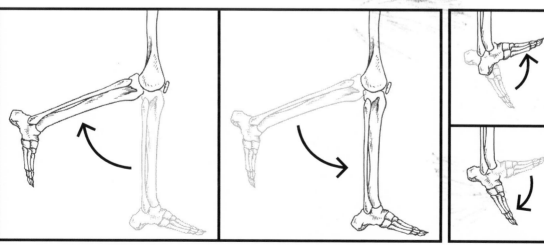

Knee: Flexion

Knee: Extension

Foot:
Dorsiflexion /
Plantar Flexion

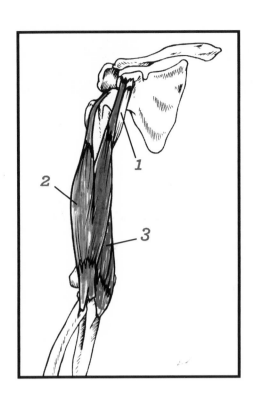

Muscles of the Musculocutaneous Nerve

BCB

1. *Coracobrachialis*
2. *Biceps Brachii*
3. *Brachialis*

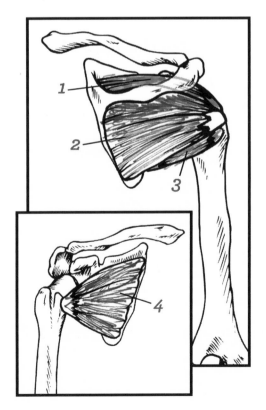

Muscles of the Rotator Cuff (S.I.T.S)

1. *Supraspinatus*
2. *Infraspinatus*
3. *Teres Minor*
4. *Subscapularis*

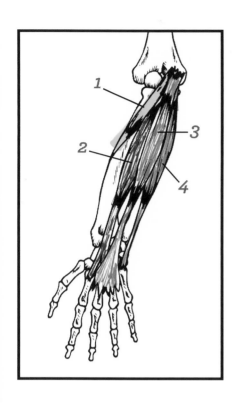

Muscles of the Common Flexor Tendon

PFPF

1. *Pronator Teres*
2. *Flexor Carpi Radialis*
3. *Palmaris*
4. *Flexor Carpi Ulnaris*

Pro Football Players Flex Up

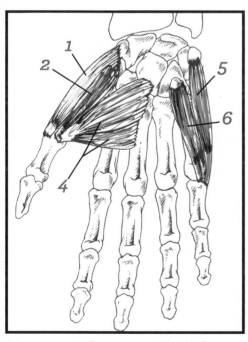

*Opponens muscles are covered by the flexors of the thumb and pinky

Thenar & Subthenar Muscles

1. *Abductor Pollicis Brevis*
2. *Flexor Pollicis Brevis*
3. *Opponens Pollicis** ~ deep
4. *Adductor Pollicis*
5. *Abductor Digiti Minimi*
6. *Flexor Digiti Minimi*
7. *Opponens Digiti Minimi** deep

½ LOAF

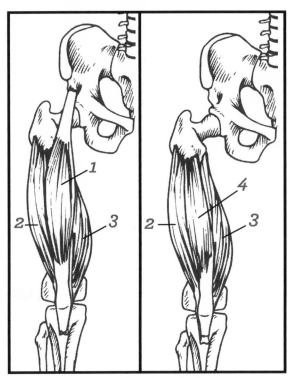

Muscles of the Quadriceps

1. *Rectus Femoris*
2. *Vastus Lateralis*
3. *Vastus Medialis*
4. *Vastus Intermedius**

*Vastus Intermedius is directly under Rectus Femoris

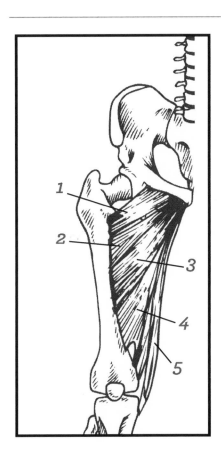

Adductor Muscles of the Thigh

1. *Pectineus*
2. *Adductor Brevis*
3. *Adductor Longus*
4. *Adductor Magnus*
5. *Gracilis*

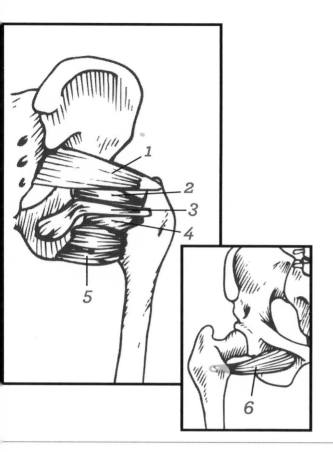

External Rotators of the Hip

1. *Piriformis*
2. *Superior Gemellus*
3. *Obturator Internus*
4. *Inferior Gemellus*
5. *Quadratus Femoris*
6. *Obturator Externus*

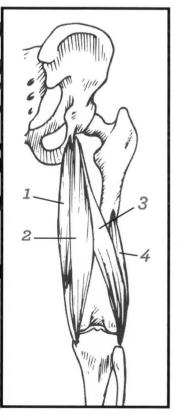

Hamstring Muscles

1. *Semitendinosus*
2. *Semimembranosus*
3. *Biceps Femoris* Long Head
4. *Biceps Femoris* Short Head

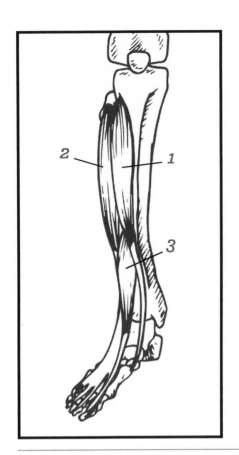

Anterior Compartment of the Leg

1. *Tibialis Anterior*

2. *Extensor Digitorum Longus*

3. *Extensor Hallucis Longus*

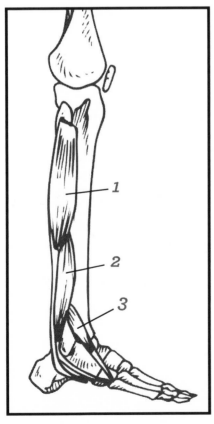

Lateral Compartment of the Leg

1. *Peroneus Longus*

2. *Peroneus Brevis*

3. *Peroneus Tertius*

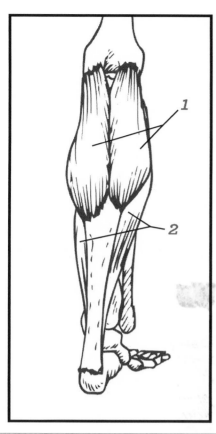

Posterior Compartment of the Leg

1. *Gastrocnemius*
2. *Soleus*

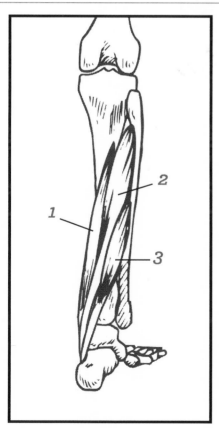

Medial Compartment of the Leg

1. *Flexor Digitorum Longus*
2. *Tibialis Posterior*
3. *Flexor Hallucis Longus*

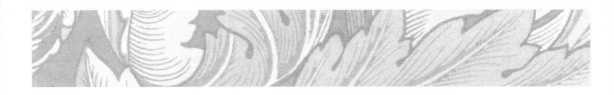

Choose individual colors for muscles based on nerve supply.

For example, if you choose light purple for the median nerve, color all muscles innervated by the median nerve in light purple. Perhaps all the radial nerve muscles will be red, and the musculocutaneous nerve muscles will be lime green! When it comes to exam time, the color of each muscle might pop into your head, making it easy to identify exactly which nerves innervate which muscles! Fill in the chart below for quick reference.

UPPER EXTREMITY

- Axillary Nerve
- CN XI
- Dorsal Scapular Nerve
- Lateral Pectoral Nerve
- Long Thoracic Nerve
- Lower Subscapular Nerve
- Medial Pectoral Nerve

- Median Nerve
- Musculocutaneous Nerve
- Nerve to Subclavius
- Radial Nerve
- Suprascapular Nerve
- Thoracodorsal Nerve
- Ulnar Nerve
- Upper Subscapular Nerve

LOWER EXTREMITY

- Deep Peroneal Nerve
- Femoral Nerve
- Inferiour Gluteal Nerve
- Lateral Plantar Nerve
- Medial Plantar Nerve
- Nerve to Obturator Intern.
- Nerve to Piriformis

- Nerve to Quadratus Fem.
- Obturator Nerve
- Sciatic- Peroneal Portion
- Sciatic- Tibial Portion
- Superficial Peroneal Nerve
- Superior Gluteal Nerve
- Tibial Nerve
- Ventral Ramus

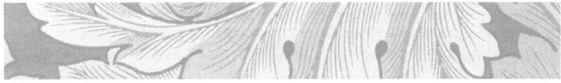

PART II:
Coloring & Labeling

Anterior Skeleton

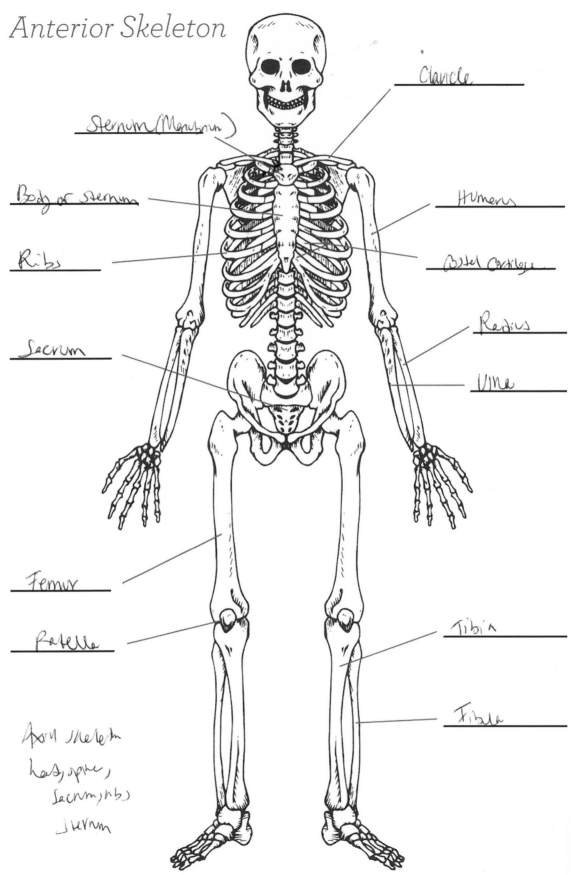

Clavicle

Sternum (Manubrium)

Body of Sternum

Ribs

Humerus

Costal Cartilage

Radius

Ulna

Sacrum

Femur

Patella

Tibia

Fibula

Axial skeleton
has, spine,
Sacrum, ribs)
Sternum

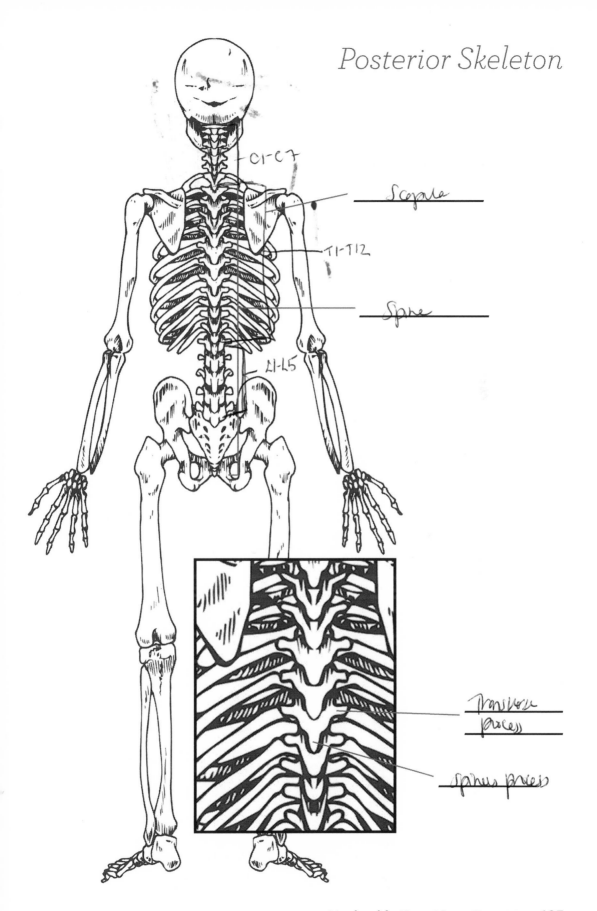

C1-C7

Scapula

T1-T12

Spine

L1-L5

Transverse process

Spinous process

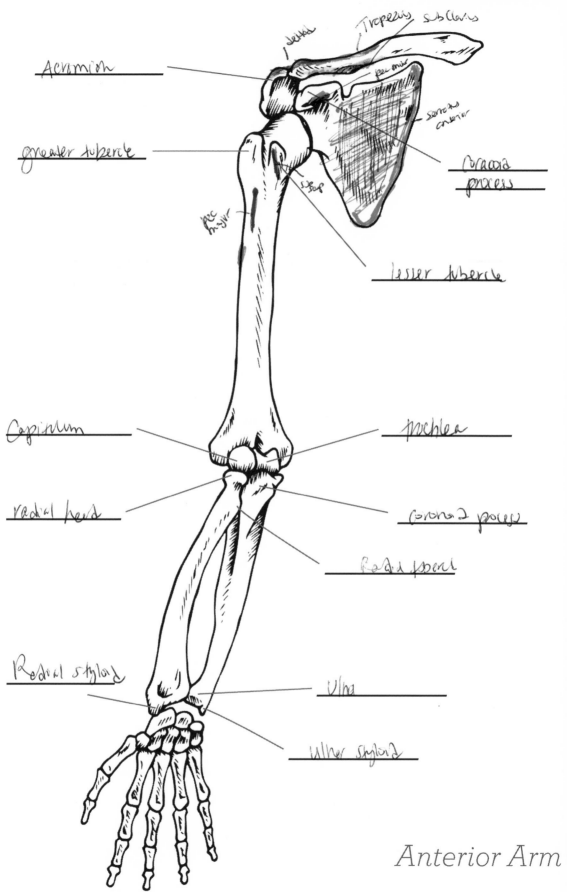

Acromion

greater tubercle

Capitulum

radial head

Radial styloid

Deltoid

Trapezius   subclavis

pec minor

serratus anterior

Coracoid process

subscap

pec major

lesser tubercle

trochlea

coronoid process

Radial tubercle

Ulna

Ulnar styloid

Anterior Arm

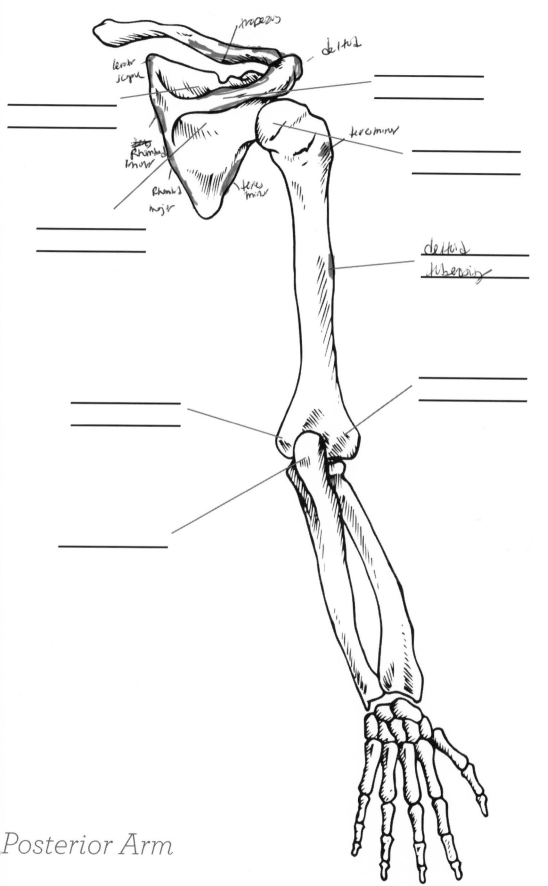

trapeus

deltid

levoto
scpu

Rhombs
minur

Rhombd
majr

tereminur

tere
minu

dettid
tuberoity

Posterior Arm

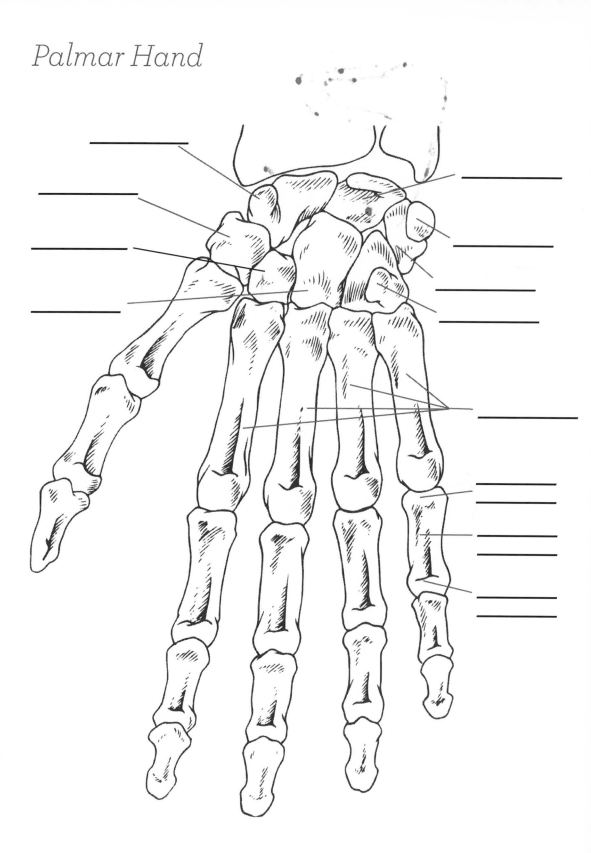

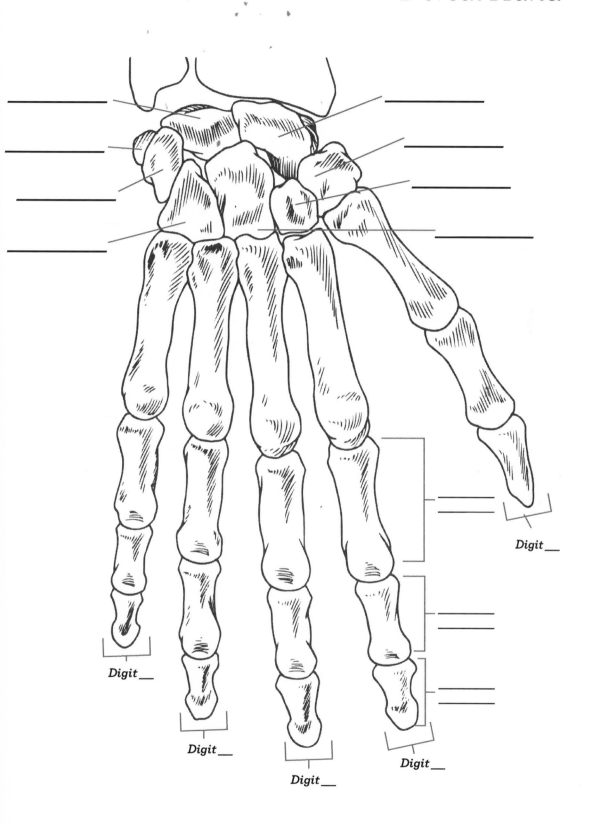

Digit __

Digit __

Digit __

Digit __

Digit __

Anterior Leg

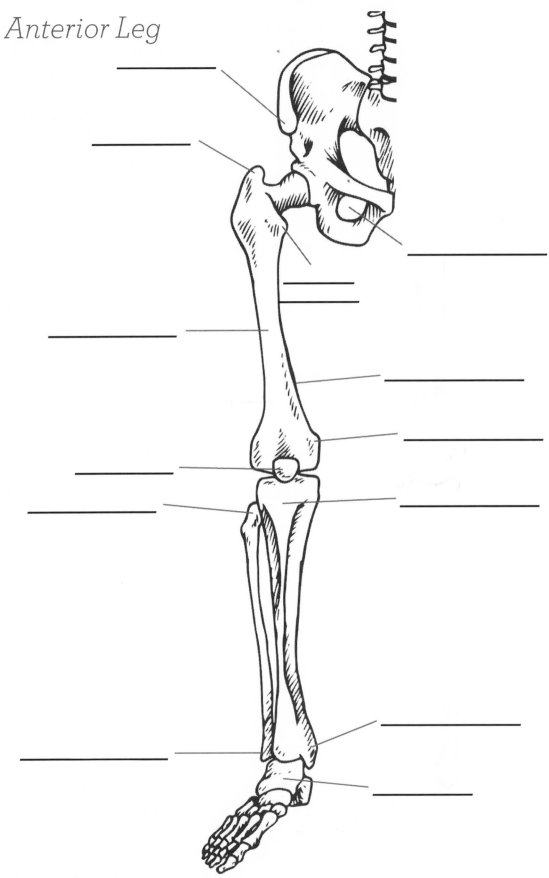

Posterior Leg

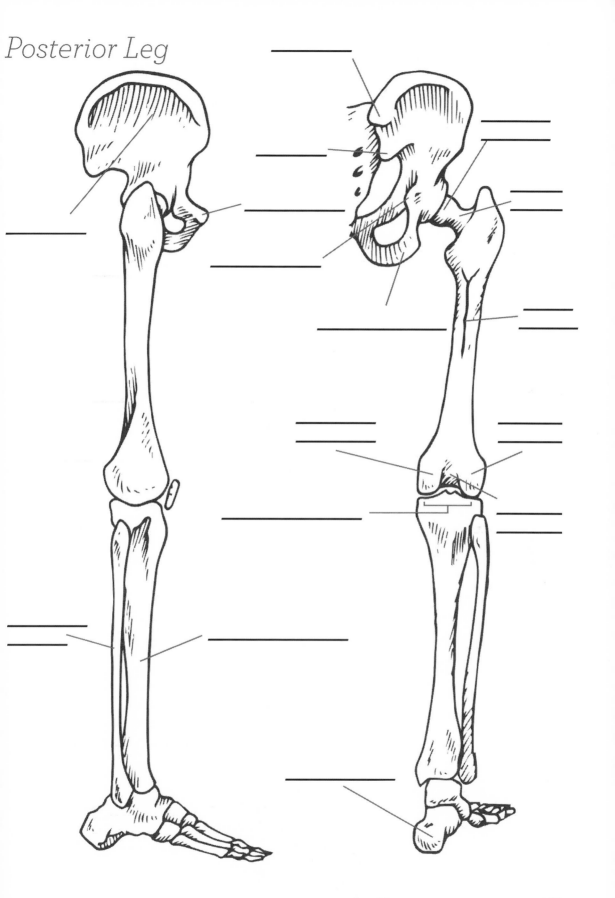

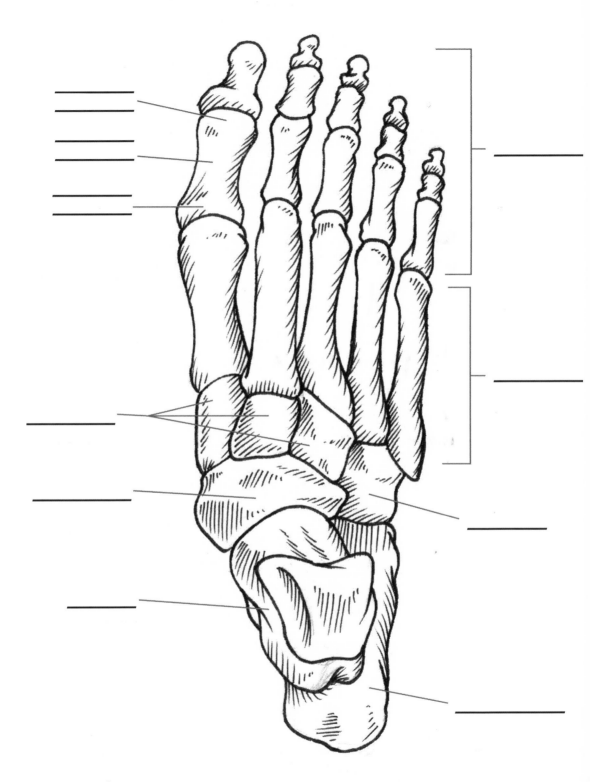

Dorsal Foot

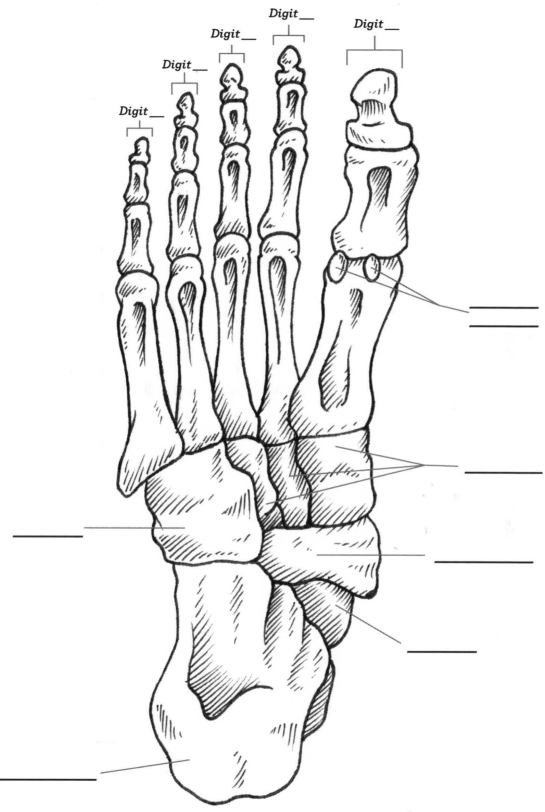

Digit __

Digit __

Digit __

Digit __

Digit __

Plantar Foot

Brachial Plexus

The brachial plexus arises from the spinal cord in the cervical spine and carries commands from the brain to the muscles and other structures, and back from those structures to the brain. The combination of nerve roots form "terminal branches." Each branch has a unique name and supplies specific muscles.

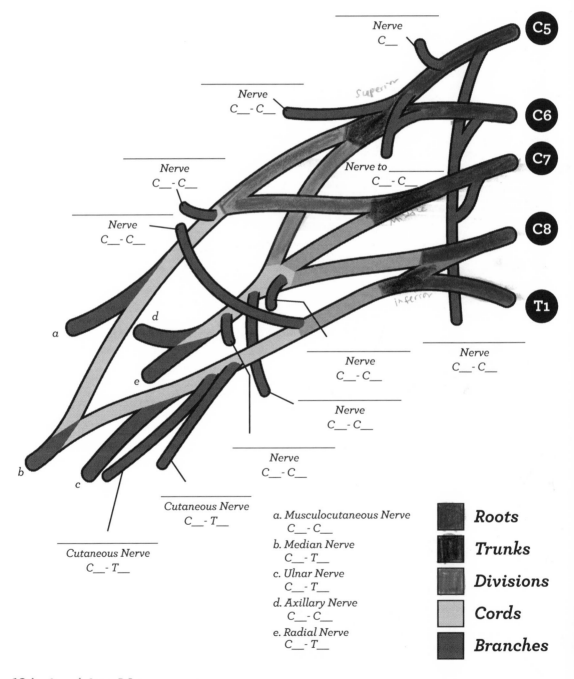

Nerve
C__

Nerve
C__ - C__

Superior

Nerve
C__ - C__

Nerve to _____
C__ - C__

Middle

Nerve
C__ - C__

Inferior

Nerve
C__ - C__

Nerve
C__ - C__

Nerve
C__ - C__

Nerve
C__ - C__

Cutaneous Nerve
C__ - T__

Cutaneous Nerve
C__ - T__

a. Musculocutaneous Nerve
  C__ - C__
b. Median Nerve
  C__ - T__
c. Ulnar Nerve
  C__ - T__
d. Axillary Nerve
  C__ - C__
e. Radial Nerve
  C__ - T__

Roots
Trunks
Divisions
Cords
Branches

Brachial Plexus

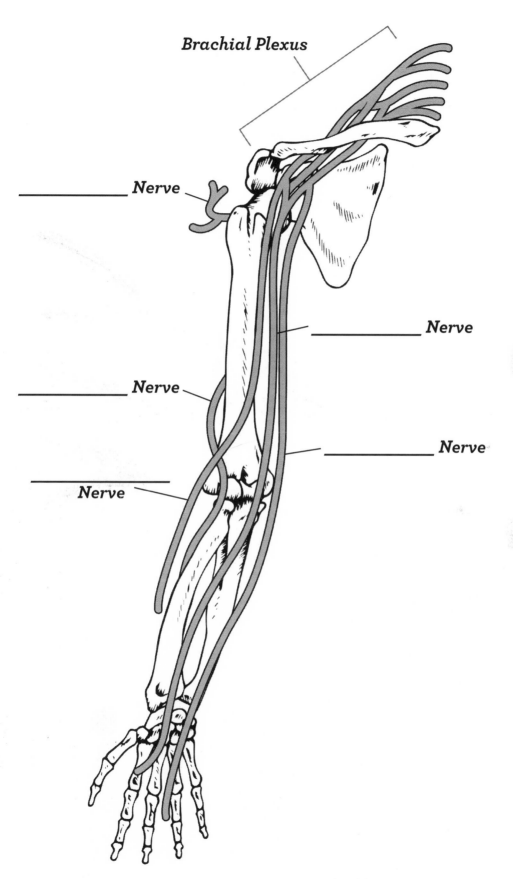

_____ **Nerve**

_____ **Nerve**

_____ **Nerve**

_____ **Nerve**

_____
Nerve

Refer to Part I and build a list of the muscles connected to each of the following nerves.

Include which nerve roots they're innervated by.

	Muscle	Nerve Roots

Axillary Nerve

Muscle	Nerve Roots
_____	_____
_____	_____

Radial Nerve

Muscle	Nerve Roots
_____	_____
_____	_____
_____	_____
_____	_____
_____	_____
_____	_____
_____	_____
_____	_____
_____	_____
_____	_____
_____	_____
_____	_____
_____	_____

Musculocutaneous Nerve

Muscle	Nerve Roots
_____	_____
_____	_____
_____	_____

Median Nerve

	Muscle	Nerve Roots
	_____	_____
	_____	_____
	_____	_____
	_____	_____
	_____	_____
	_____	_____
	_____	_____
	_____	_____
	_____	_____
	_____	_____

Ulnar Nerve

_____	_____
_____	_____
_____	_____
_____	_____
_____	_____
_____	_____
_____	_____
_____	_____
_____	_____
_____	_____

Lumbar Plexus

Like the Brachial Plexus, the Lumbar Plexus gives rise to a
number of large nerves that supplies muscles of the lower extremity,
low abdomen and pelvic bowl.

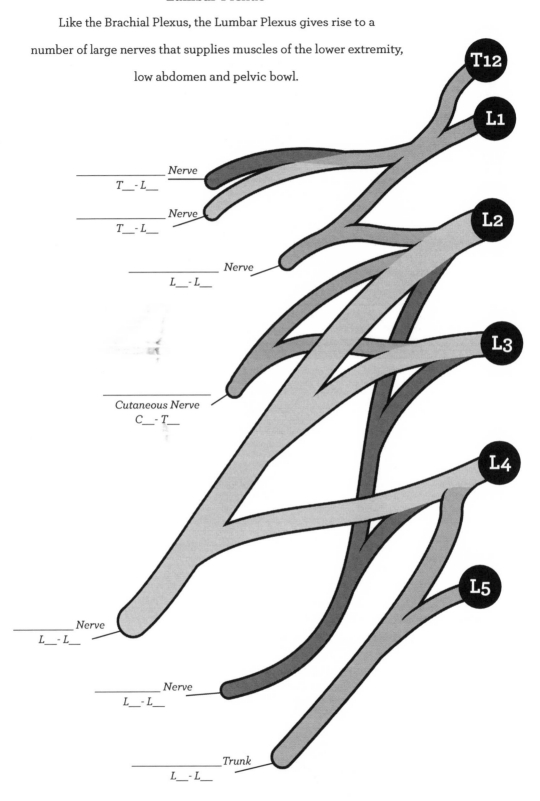

_____ _Nerve_
T___- L___

_____ _Nerve_
T___- L___

_____ _Nerve_
L___- L___

_____
Cutaneous Nerve
C___- T___

_____ _Nerve_
L___- L___

_____ _Nerve_
L___- L___

_____ _Trunk_
L___- L___

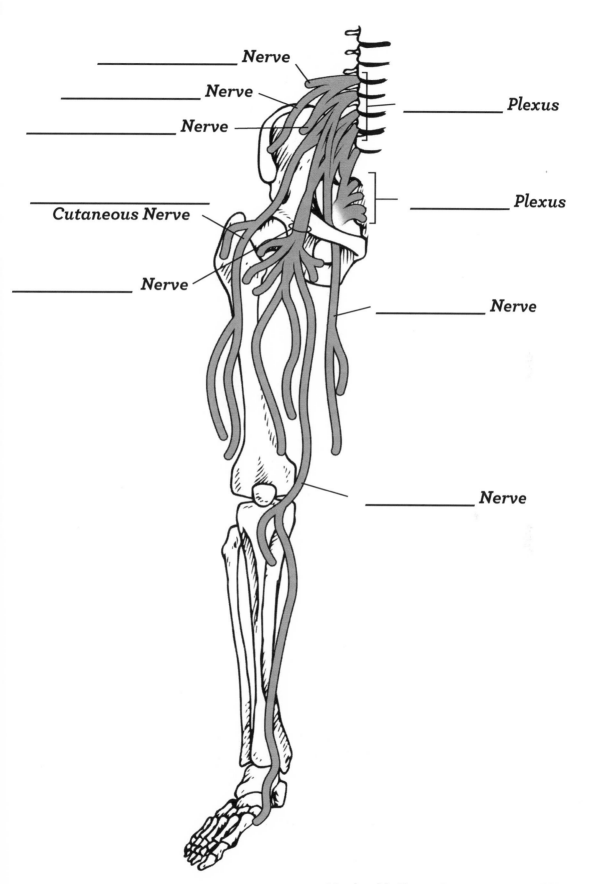

_____ *Nerve*

_____ *Nerve*

_____ *Nerve*

_____ *Cutaneous Nerve*

_____ *Nerve*

_____ *Plexus*

_____ *Plexus*

_____ *Nerve*

_____ *Nerve*

Sacral Plexus

The Sacral Plexus works in harmony with the Lumbar plexus to innervate the lower extremity. While the Lumbar Plexus supplies mainly the ventromedial thigh, the sacral plexus controls the dorsolateral portion.

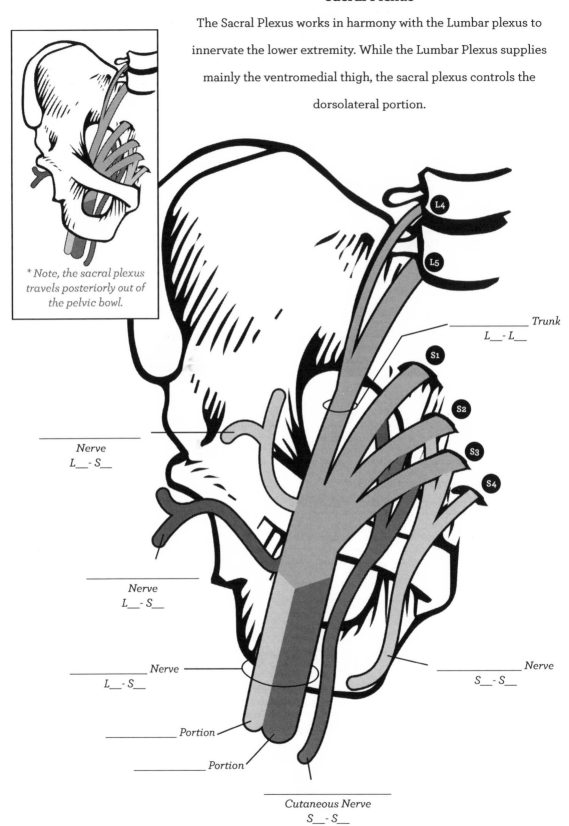

* Note, the sacral plexus travels posteriorly out of the pelvic bowl.

L4

L5

S1

S2

S3

S4

_____ *Trunk*
L___ - L___

_____
Nerve
L___ - S___

_____
Nerve
L___ - S___

_____ *Nerve*
L___ - S___

_____ *Nerve*
S___ - S___

_____ *Portion*

_____ *Portion*

_____
Cutaneous Nerve
S___ - S___

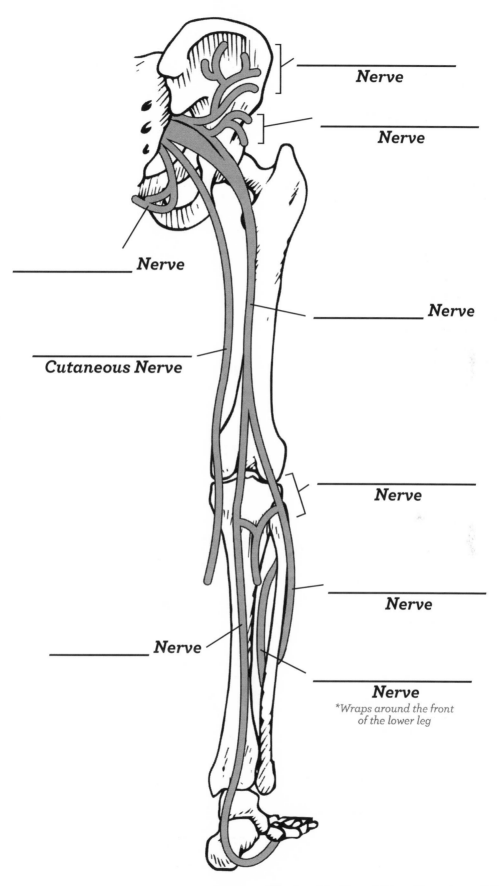

Nerve

Nerve

Nerve

Nerve

Cutaneous Nerve

Nerve

Nerve

Nerve

Nerve
*Wraps around the front
of the lower leg*

Refer to Part I and build a list of the muscles connected to each of the following nerves.

Include which nerve roots they're innervated by.

	Muscle	Nerve Roots

Femoral Nerve

Obturator Nerve

Inferior Gluteal Nerve

Superior Gluteal Nerve

Muscle	Nerve Roots
_____	_____
_____	_____
_____	_____

Sciatic Nerve

Muscle	Nerve Roots
_____	_____
_____	_____
_____	_____
_____	_____

Tibial Nerve

Muscle	Nerve Roots
_____	_____
_____	_____
_____	_____
_____	_____
_____	_____
_____	_____
_____	_____
_____	_____

Superficial Peroneal Nerve

_____ _____

_____ _____

Deep Peroneal Nerve

_____ _____

_____ _____

_____ _____

_____ _____

_____ _____

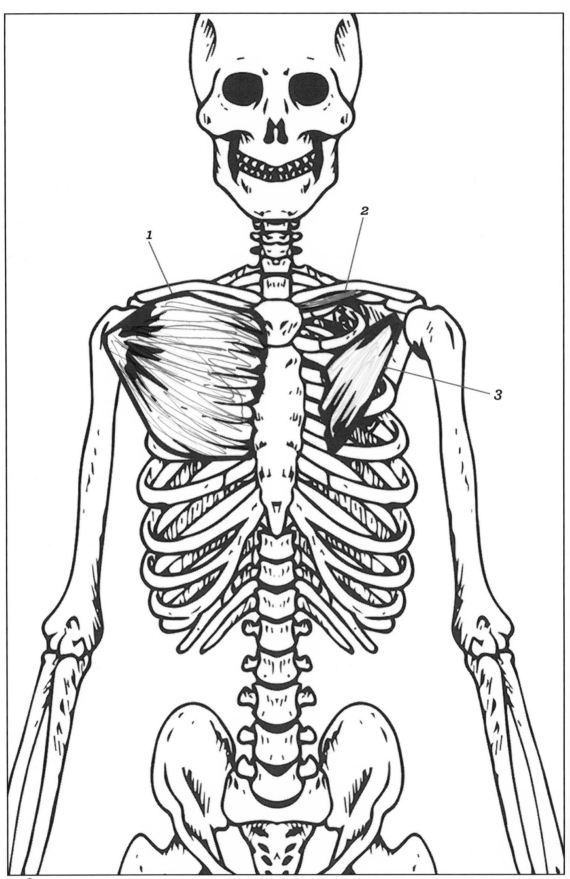

1. Pectoralis Major

Origin: _Clavicle, Costal cartilage, sternum_

Insertion: _Lateral lip bicipital groove_

Innervation: _Medial/lateral pectoral_

Blood Supply: _____

Function: _Shoulder protraction, internal rotation + adduction_

2. Subclavius

Origin: _Rib 1_

Insertion: _Mid Clavicle_

Innervation: _Subclavius_

Blood Supply: _____

Function: _Rib cage elevation, scapula anterior + inferior_

3. Pectoralis Minor

Origin: _ribs 3-5_

Insertion: _Coracoid process_

Innervation: _Medial pectoral_

Blood Supply: _____

Function: _Scapula protraction + elevation_

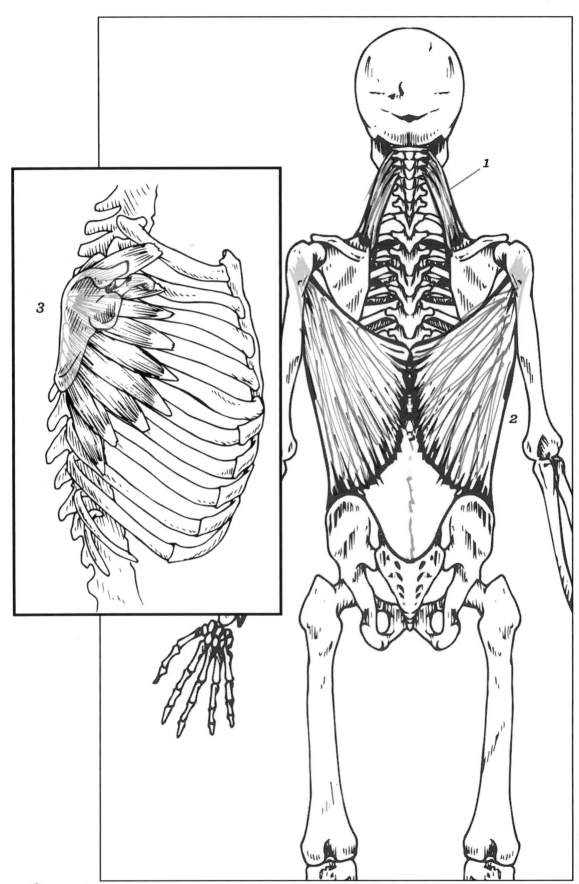

1. Levator Scapulae

Origin: C1- C4 transverse process

Insertion: Medial superior border scapula

Innervation: dorsal scapula

Blood Supply: _____

Function: Scapular elevation

2. Latissimus Dorsi

T7 *5* *Lady between 2 majors*

Origin: T7-L5 spinous process, iliac crest, fascia, low 3 ribs

Insertion: Medial lip bicipital groove

Innervation: thoracodorsal nerve

Blood Supply: _____

Function: internal rotation, extension, adduction

3. Serratus Anterior

9 feathers in your cap

Origin: lateral aspect ribs 1-9

Insertion: Medial border scapula

Innervation: long thoracic C5-7

Blood Supply: _____

Function: Scapula protraction

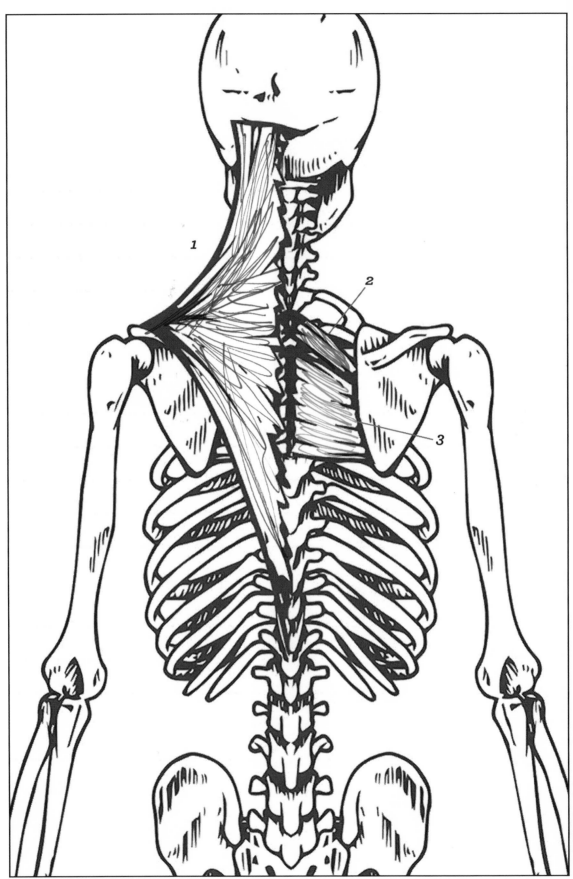

1. Trapezius

Origin: _External occipital protuberance, spinous process C1-T12, Nuchal ligament_

Insertion: _Clavicle, Spine of scapula_

Innervation: _CN XI + Ventral Rami_

Blood Supply: _____

Function: _Scapula retraction/depression, extend head + neck_

2. Rhomboid Minor

Origin: _C7-T1 spinous process_

Insertion: _medial border Scapula_

Innervation: _dorsal scapular nerve_

Blood Supply: _____

Function: _elevation, retraction + rotation_

3. Rhomboid Major

Origin: _T2-T5 spinous process_

Insertion: _Medial border scapula_

Innervation: _dorsal scapular nerve C5_

Blood Supply: _____

Function: _elevation, retraction + rotation_

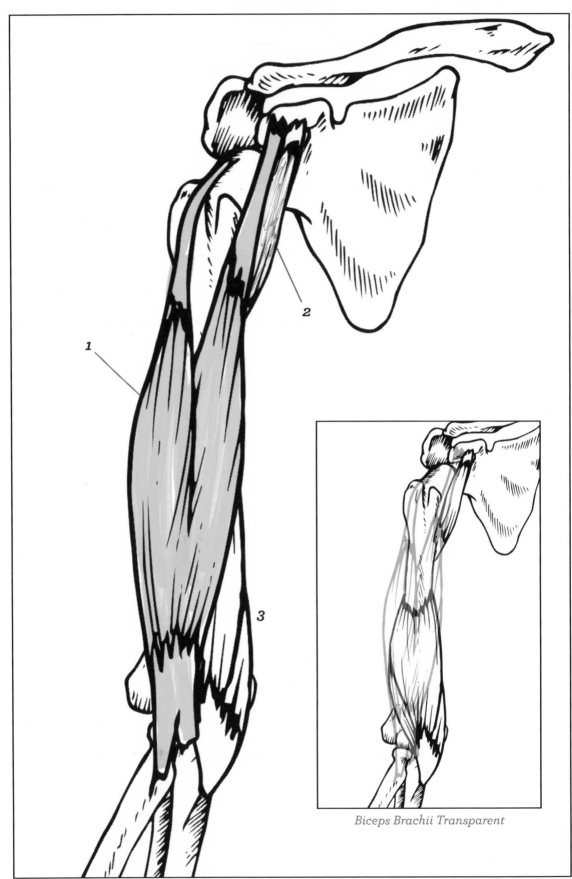

Biceps Brachii Transparent

1. Biceps Brachii

Origin: _Supraglenoid tubercle + Coracoid process_

Insertion: _radial tuberosity, bicipital aponeurosis_

Innervation: _Musculocutaneous C5-6_

Blood Supply: _____

Function: _Elbow flexion, supination, shoulder flexion_

2. Coracobrachialis

Origin: _Coracoid process_

Insertion: _lateral humerus_

Innervation: _Musculocutaneous C5-7_

Blood Supply: _____

Function: _Shoulder adduction, flexion_

3. Brachialis

Origin: _lower humerus_

Insertion: _coronoid process ulna_

Innervation: _Musculocutaneous C5-7_

Blood Supply: _____

Function: _elbow flexion_

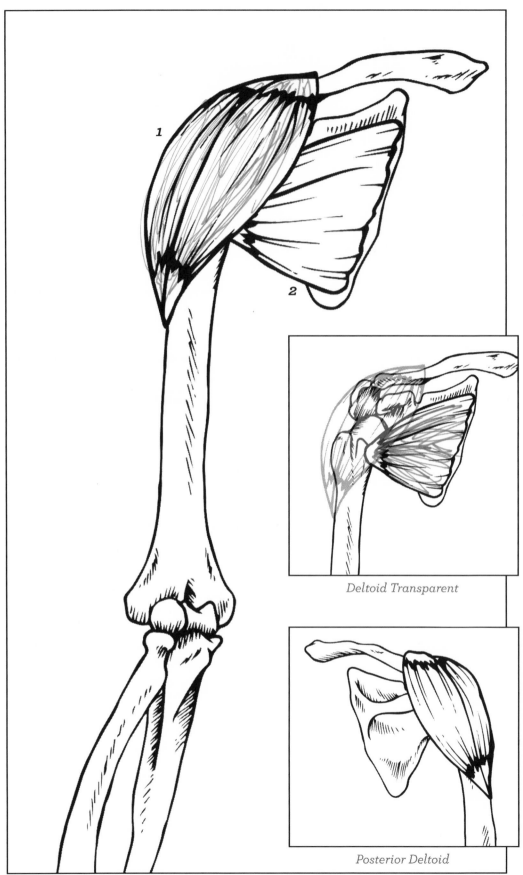

Deltoid Transparent

Posterior Deltoid

1. Deltoid

Origin: _Clavicle, Acromion process, spine of scapula_

Insertion: _deltoid tuberosity_

Innervation: _Axillary C5-6_

Blood Supply: _____

Function: _shoulder flexion, abduction, extension_

2. Subscapularis

Origin: _Subscapular fossa_

Insertion: _lesser tubercle_

Innervation: _Subscapular upper + lower nerve_

Blood Supply: _____

Function: _internal rotation, humeral stabilization_

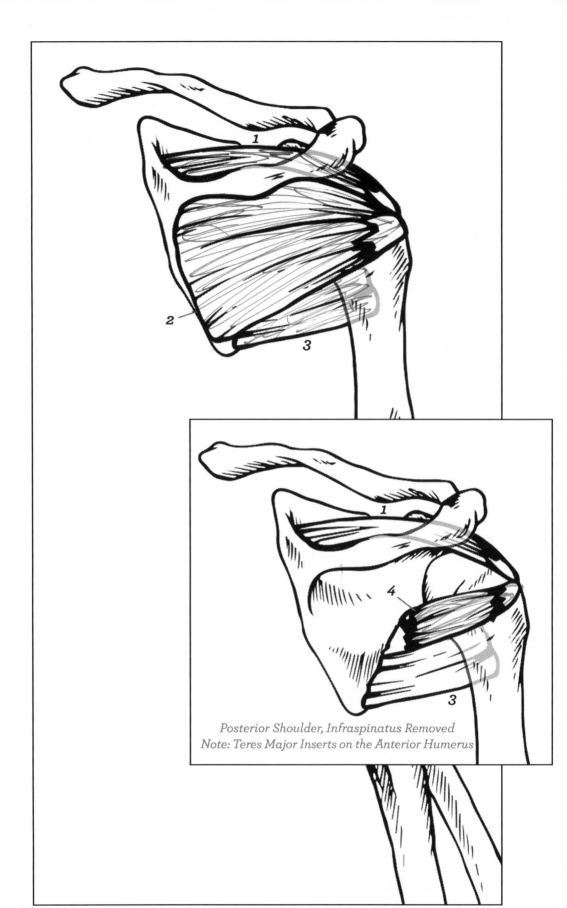

Posterior Shoulder, Infraspinatus Removed
Note: Teres Major Inserts on the Anterior Humerus

1. Supraspinatus

Origin: _Suprascapular fossa_

Insertion: _greater tuberosity_

Innervation: ~~30° abduct~~ _Suprascapular C5-C6_

Blood Supply: _____

Function: _30° shoulder abduction, humeral stabilization_

2. Infraspinatus

Origin: _infraspinatus fossa_

Insertion: _greater tuberosity_

Innervation: _Suprascapular C5-C6_

Blood Supply: _____

Function: _external rotation, humeral stabilization_

3. Teres Major

Origin: _inferior angle scapula_

Insertion: _medial lip bicipital groove_

Innervation: _lower subscapular nerve C5-C6_

Blood Supply: _____

Function: _internal rotation, adduction, extension_

4. Teres Minor

Origin: _lateral border scapula_

Insertion: _Greater tuberosity_

Innervation: _posterior axillary nerve C5-C6_

Blood Supply: _____

Function: _external rotation, humeral stabilization_

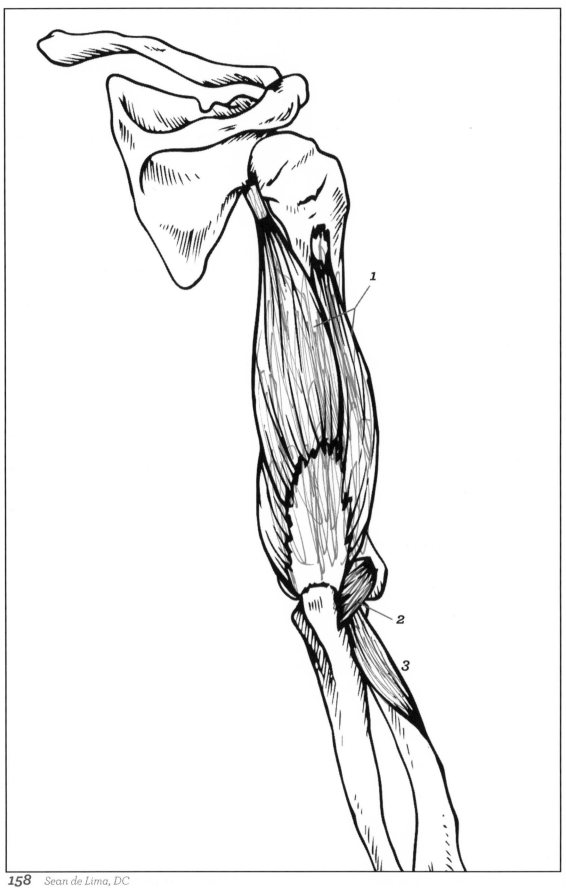

1. Triceps Brachii

Origin: _infraglenoid tuberole dorsal humerus upper +lower_

Insertion: _Olecranon process_

_____

Innervation: _radial nerve (6-8_

Blood Supply: _____

Function: _elbow extension_

2. Anconeus

Origin: _lateral epicondyle_

Insertion: _Olecranon process_

Innervation: _radial nerve (6 -8_

Blood Supply: _____

Function: _elbow extension_

3. Supinator

Origin: _Lateral epicondyle_

Insertion: _radial shaft_

Innervation: _Radial nerve deep (c5-c6)_

Blood Supply: _____

Function: _Supination_

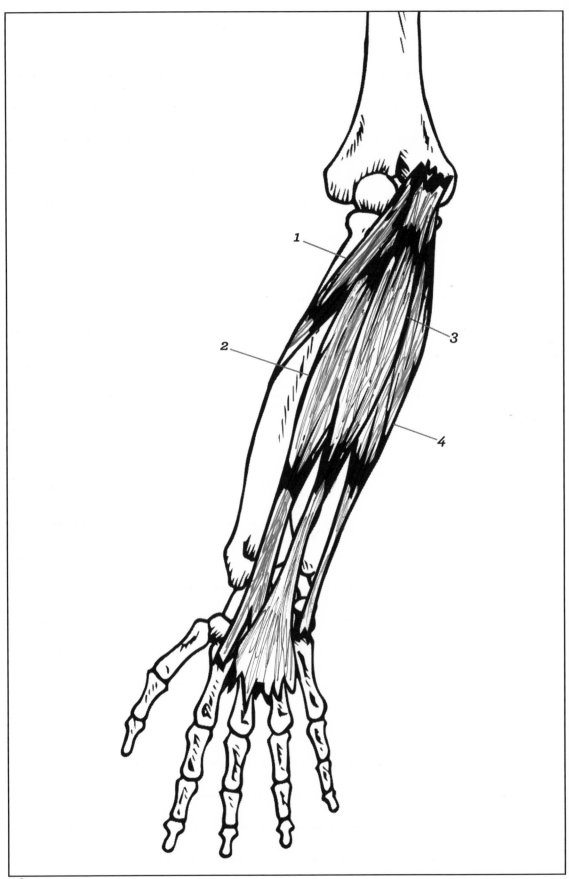

1. Pronator Teres

☐

Origin: Medial supracondylar ridge

Insertion: Lateral radius

Innervation: Median nerve (C6-7

Blood Supply: _____

Function: pronation

2. Flexor Carpi Radialis

☐

Origin: Common flexor tendon - medial epicondyle

Insertion: base 2nd + 3rd Metacarpal

Innervation: Median nerve C6-8

Blood Supply: _____

Function: Flex + radial deviate wrist

3. Palmaris Longus

☐

Origin: Common flexor tendon : medial epicondyle

Insertion: palmar aponeurosis

Innervation: Median (C7-T1)

Blood Supply: _____

Function: assist wrist flexion

4. Flexor Carpi Ulnaris

☐

Origin: Common flexor tendon : medial epicondyle

Insertion: 5th metacarpal + pisiform.

Innervation: Ulnar nerve C7-C8

Blood Supply: _____

Function: Flex + ulnar deviate wrist

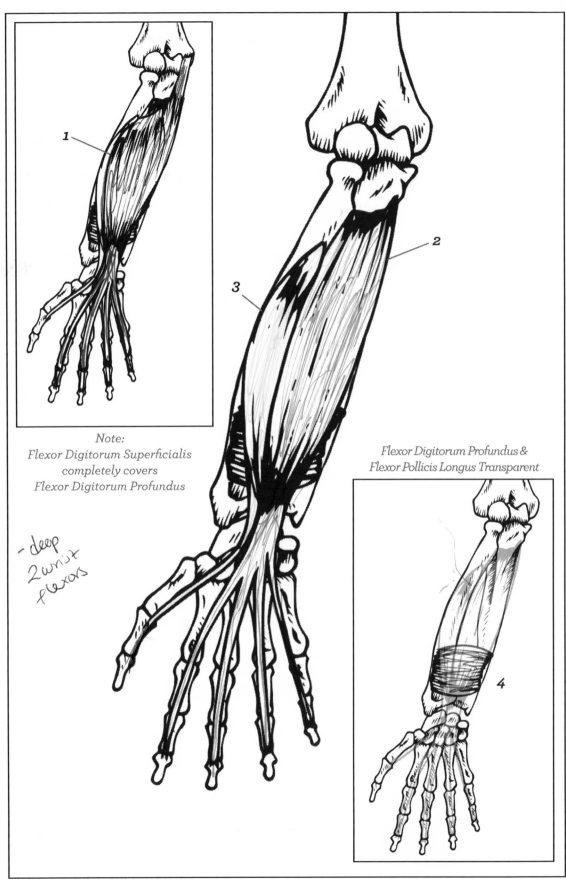

Note:
*Flexor Digitorum Superficialis
completely covers
Flexor Digitorum Profundus*

*Flexor Digitorum Profundus &
Flexor Pollicis Longus Transparent*

- deep
2 wrist
flexors

1. Flexor Digitorum Superficialis

Origin: Common flexor tendon + proximal ulna + radius

Insertion: As 2 slips into base of middle phalanges

Innervation: Median nerve C7-T1

Blood Supply: _____

Function: Finger flexion @ PIP assists MCPs + wrist

2. Flexor Digitorum Profundus

Origin: proximal ulna ; Anterior interosseous membrane

Insertion: base of distal phalanges 2-5

Innervation: Median (radial half C8T1) + ulnar (ulnar half C8-T1)

Blood Supply: _____

Function: Finger flexion DIPs assists, PIPs, MCPs + wrist

3. Flexor Pollicis Longus

Origin: Radius proximal ; interosseous membrane

Insertion: base of distal phalanx

Innervation: Median C7-T1

Blood Supply: _____

Function: Thumb flexion

4. Pronator Quadratus

Origin: distal ulna

Insertion: distal radius

Innervation: Median C7-T1

Blood Supply: _____

Function: pronation

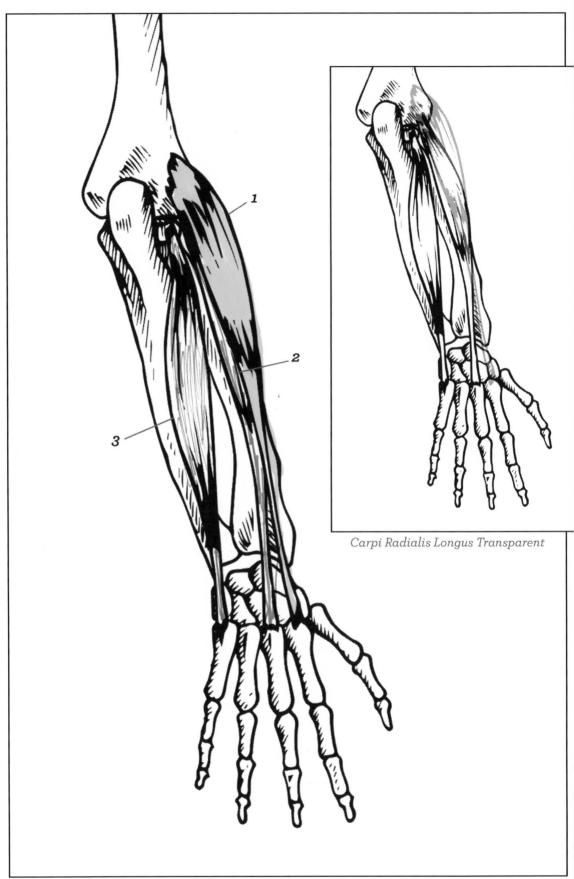

Carpi Radialis Longus Transparent

1. Extensor Carpi Radialis Longus

Origin: _Common extensor tendon: Lateral epicondyle_

Insertion: _base of 2nd Metacarpal_

Innervation: _Radial nerve C6-7_

Blood Supply: _____

Function: _Wrist extension + radial deviation_

2. Extensor Carpi Radialis Brevis

Origin: _common extensor tendon: Lateral epicondyle_

Insertion: _base of 3rd metacarpel_

Innervation: _Radial nerve deep branch C6-7_

Blood Supply: _____

Function: _Wrist extension + radial deviation_

3. Extensor Carpi Ulnaris

Origin: _Common extensor tendon: Lateral epicondyle_

Insertion: _base of 5th metacarpal_

Innervation: _Radial nerve deep branch C6-7_

Blood Supply: _____

Function: _Wrist extension + ulnar deviation_

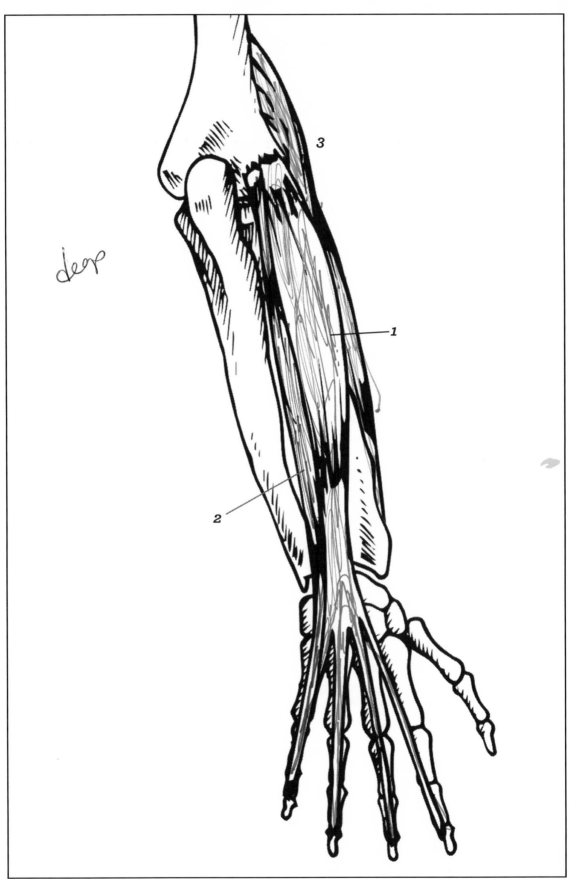

deep

3

1

2

1. Extensor Digitorum

Origin: Common extensor tendon; lateral epicondyle

Insertion: Extensor expansion middle + distal phalanges

Innervation: Radial nerve PIN C6-8

Blood Supply:

Function: Extend digits 2-5

2. Extensor Digiti Minimi

Origin: Common extensor tendon; lateral epicondyle

Insertion: Extensor expansion 5th digit

Innervation: Radial nerve PIN C6-C8

Blood Supply:

Function: Extend 5th digit

3. Brachioradialis

Origin: Supracondylar ridge / lateral epicondyle

Insertion: Radial styloid

Innervation: Radial nerve C5-6

Blood Supply:

Function: elbow flexion

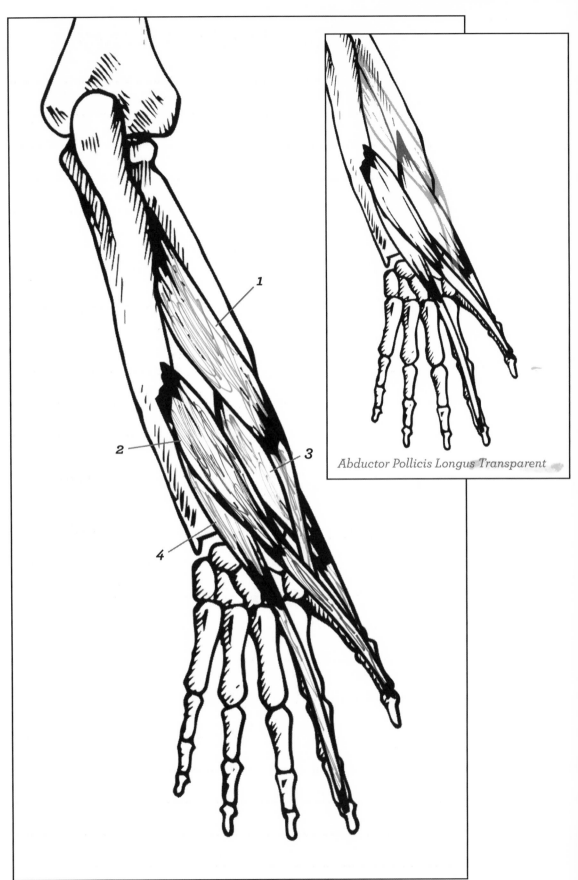

Abductor Pollicis Longus Transparent

1. Abductor Pollicis Longus

Origin: _proximal ulna, radius, interosseous membrane_

Insertion: _lateral base of 1st Metacarpel_

Innervation: _Radial nerve PIN C6-8_

Blood Supply: _____

Function: _Thumb abduction/extension_

2. Extensor Pollicis Longus

Origin: _Radius + interosseous membrane_

Insertion: _Distal phalanx 1st digit_

Innervation: _Radial nerve -PIN C6-8_

Blood Supply: _____

Function: _Extension thumb_

3. Extensor Pollicis Brevis

Origin: _Mid ulna + interosseous membrane_

Insertion: _base of phalanx 1_

Innervation: _Radial nerve -PIN C6-8_

Blood Supply: _____

Function: _Extension thumb MCP_

4. Extensor Indicis

Origin: _Ulna + interosseous membrane_

Insertion: _extensor expansion index finger_

Innervation: _Radial nerve PIN C6-8_

Blood Supply: _____

Function: _index finger extension_

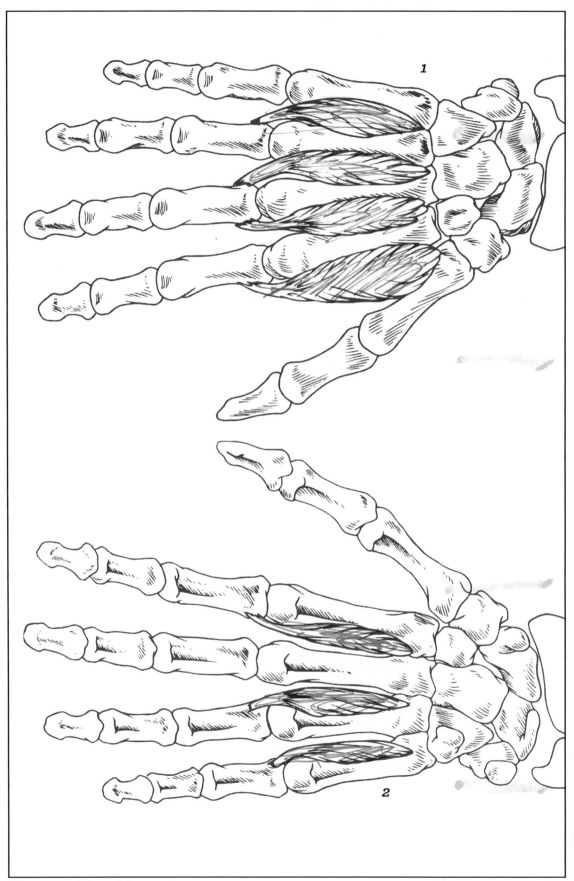

1. Dorsal Interossei

Origin: _Adjacent metacarpals_

Insertion: _proximal phalanx 2-4 extensor expansion_

Innervation: _Ulnar deep branch_

Blood Supply: _____

Function: _digit Abduction_

2. Palmar Interossei

Origin: _Metacarpals 2,4,5_

Insertion: _Corresponding proximal phalanx_

Innervation: _Ulnar deep branch_

Blood Supply: _____

Function: _digit adduction_

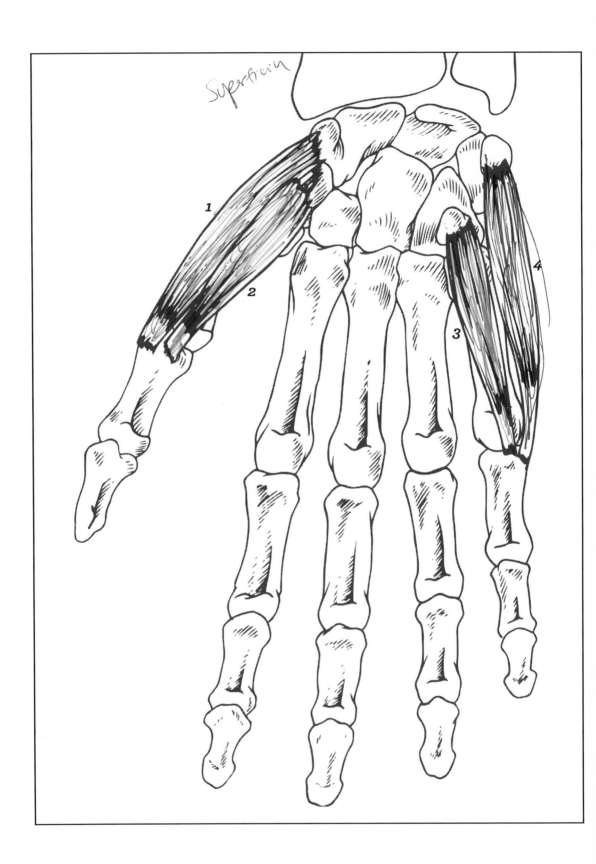

Superficial

½ LUAF

1. Abductor Pollicis Brevis

Origin: Scaphoid + trapezium

Insertion: Radial proximal phalanx

Innervation: Median nerve recurrent branch

Blood Supply: _____

Function: Thumb abduction

2. Flexor Pollicis Brevis

Origin: Trapezium + flexor retinaculum

Insertion: proximal phalanx

Innervation: _____

Blood Supply: Flex medial head - deep ulnar, median recurrent

Function: Flex MCP thumb

3. Flexor Digiti Minimi

Origin: hook hamate

Insertion: Volar P1

Innervation: Ulnar nerve

Blood Supply: _____

Function: Flex MCP 5F

4. Abductor Digiti Minimi

Origin: pisiform

Insertion: Ulnar proximal phalanx

Innervation: Ulnar nerve deep

Blood Supply: _____

Function: Abduct 5F

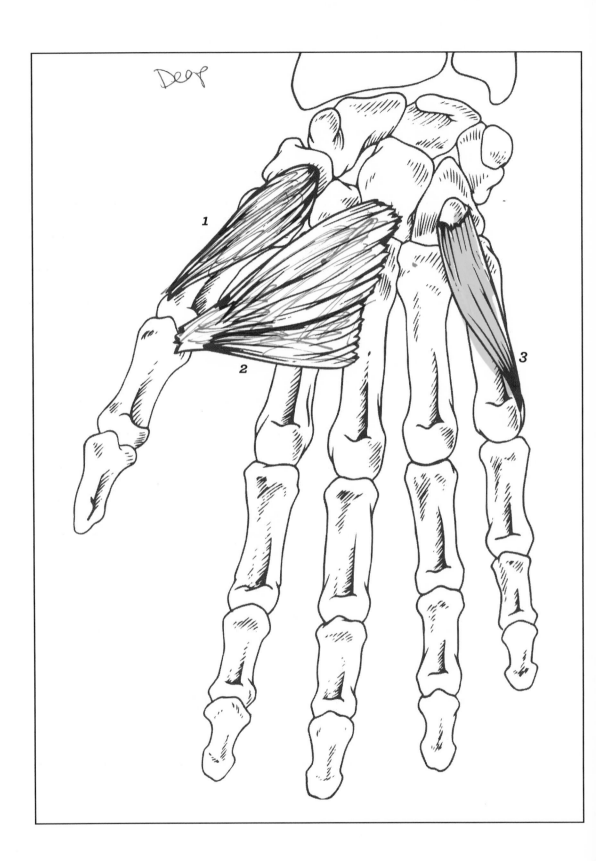

Deep

1

2

3

1. Opponens Pollicis

Origin: _Trapezium_

Insertion: _Radial 1st metacarpal_

Innervation: _Median recurrent branch_

Blood Supply: _____

Function: _thumb opposition_

2. Adductor Pollicis

Origin: _1st + 2nd metacarpal, trapezoid, Capitate_

Insertion: _Medial side proximal phalanx_

Innervation: _Ulnar nerve - deep branch_

Blood Supply: _____

Function: _thumb adduction_

3. Opponens Digiti Minimi

Origin: _hook of hamate_

Insertion: _Medial 5th metacarpal_

Innervation: _Ulnar nerve - deep branch_

Blood Supply: _____

Function: _SF opposition_

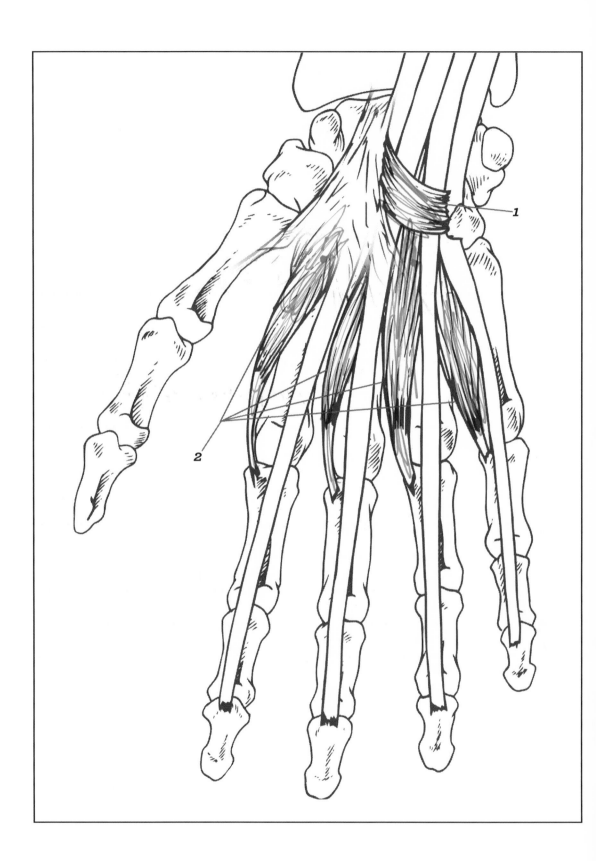

1. Palmaris Brevis

Origin: Flexor retinaculum + palmar aponeurosis

Insertion: Skin of palm

Innervation: Ulnar nerve

Blood Supply: _____

Function: pull on skin hypothenar eminence

2. Lumbricals

Origin: tendons of FDP

Insertion: Ext expansion of digits 2-5

Innervation: 1st+2nd lumbricals median   3+4th Ulnar nerve

Blood Supply: _____

Function: Flexion of MCP + extension IPs

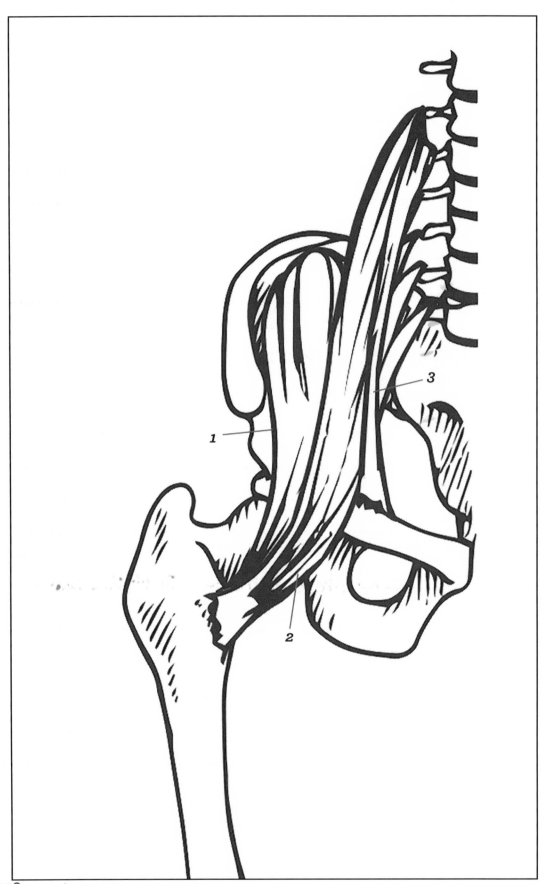

1. Iliacus

Origin: _____

Insertion: _____

Innervation: _____

Blood Supply: _____

Function: _____

2. Psoas Major

Origin: _____

Insertion: _____

Innervation: _____

Blood Supply: _____

Function: _____

3. Psoas Minor

Origin: _____

Insertion: _____

Innervation: _____

Blood Supply: _____

Function: _____

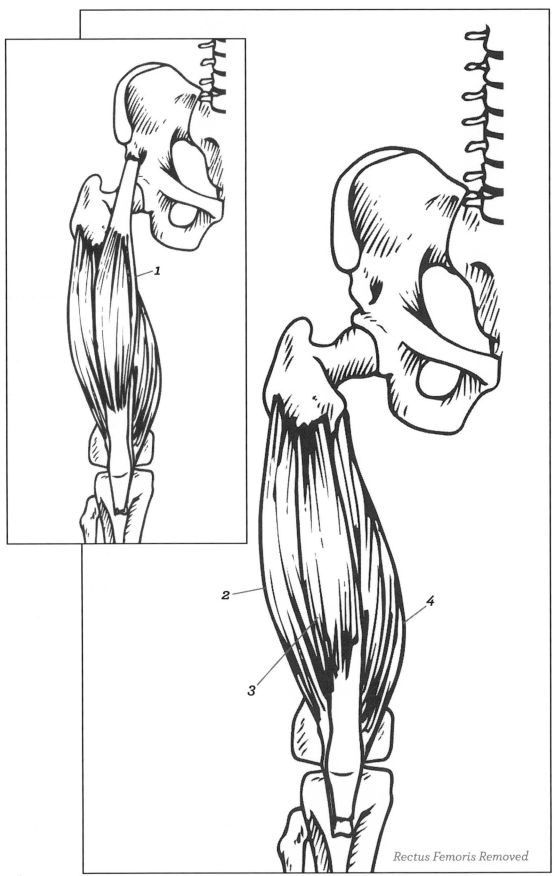

Rectus Femoris Removed

1. Rectus Femoris

Origin: _____

Insertion: _____

Innervation: _____

Blood Supply: _____

Function: _____

2. Vastus Lateralis

Origin: _____

Insertion: _____

Innervation: _____

Blood Supply: _____

Function: _____

3. Vastus Intermedius

Origin: _____

Insertion: _____

Innervation: _____

Blood Supply: _____

Function: _____

4. Vastus Medialis

Origin: _____

Insertion: _____

Innervation: _____

Blood Supply: _____

Function: _____

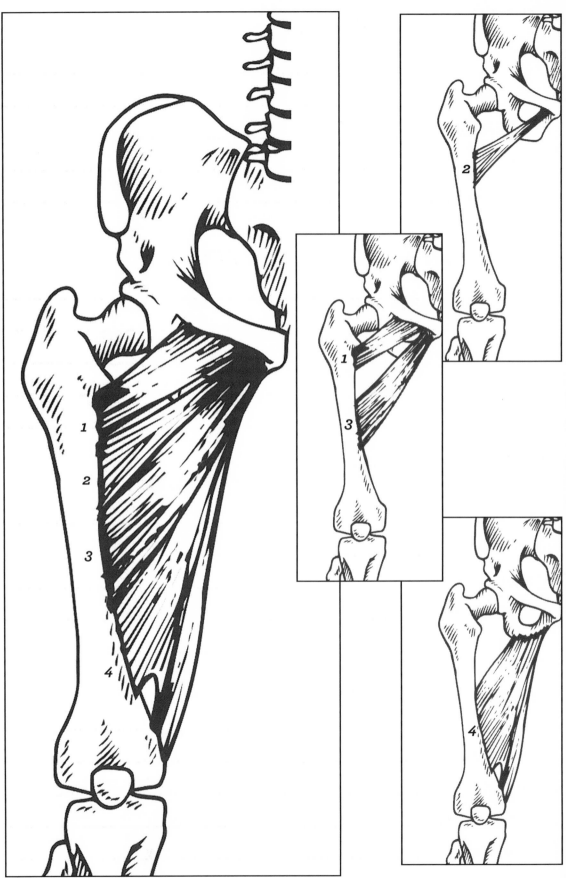

1. Pectineus

Origin: _____

Insertion: _____

Innervation: _____

Blood Supply: _____

Function: _____

2. Adductor Brevis

Origin: _____

Insertion: _____

Innervation: _____

Blood Supply: _____

Function: _____

3. Adductor Longus

Origin: _____

Insertion: _____

Innervation: _____

Blood Supply: _____

Function: _____

4. Adductor Magnus

Origin: _____

Insertion: _____

Innervation: _____

Blood Supply: _____

Function: _____

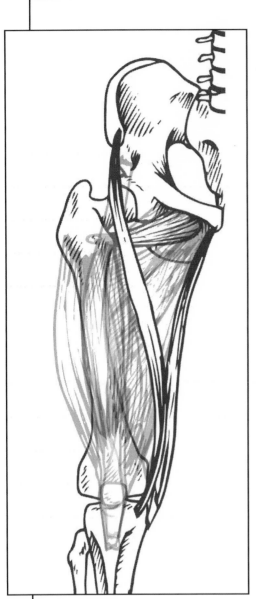

*In relation to the Quadricep and
Abductor groups*

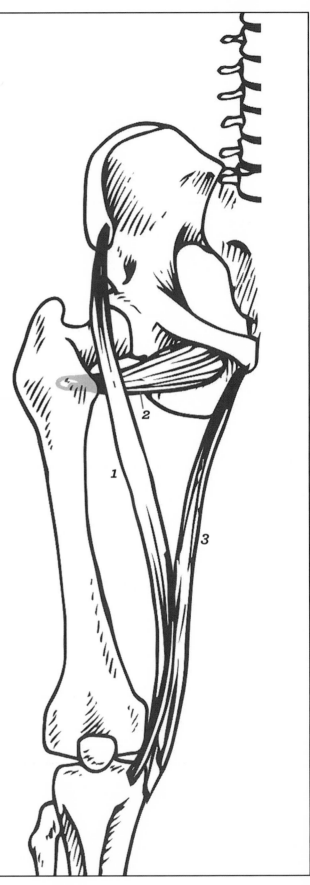

1. Sartorius

Origin: _____

Insertion: _____

Innervation: _____

Blood Supply: _____

Function: _____

2. Obturator Externus

Origin: _____

Insertion: _____

Innervation: _____

Blood Supply: _____

Function: _____

3. Gracilis

Origin: _____

Insertion: _____

Innervation: _____

Blood Supply: _____

Function: _____

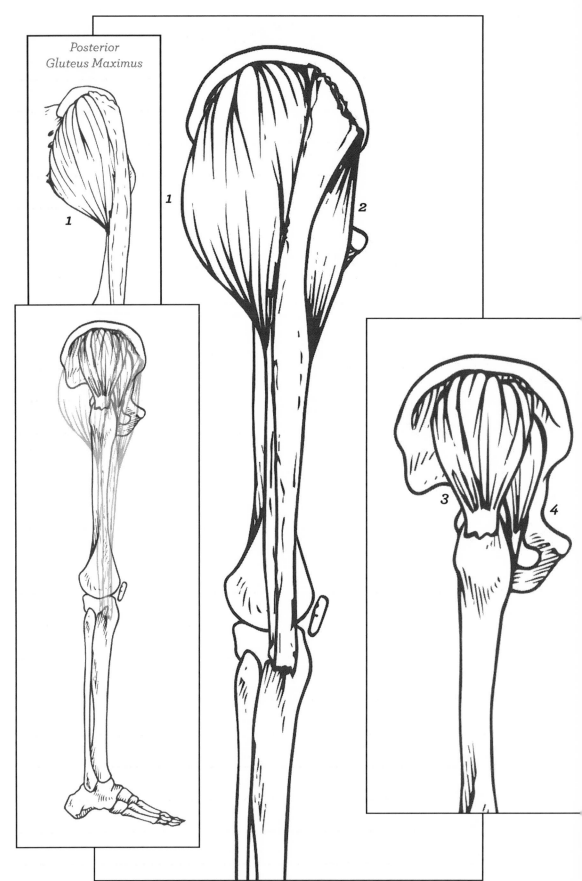

Posterior
Gluteus Maximus

1. Gluteus Maximus

Origin: _____

Insertion: _____

Innervation: _____

Blood Supply: _____

Function: _____

2. Tensor Fascia Latae

Origin: _____

Insertion: _____

Innervation: _____

Blood Supply: _____

Function: _____

3. Gluteus Medius

Origin: _____

Insertion: _____

Innervation: _____

Blood Supply: _____

Function: _____

4. Gluteus Minimus

Origin: _____

Insertion: _____

Innervation: _____

Blood Supply: _____

Function: _____

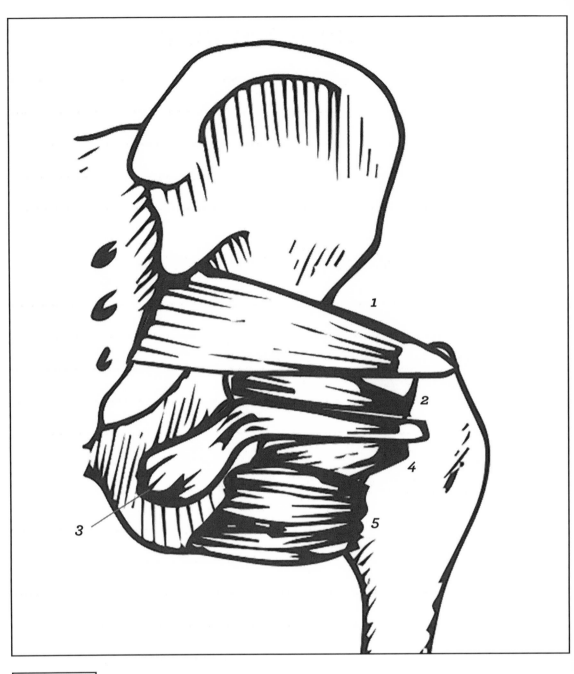

1. Piriformis

Origin: _____

Insertion: _____

Innervation: _____

Blood Supply: _____

Function: _____

2. Superior Gemellus

Origin: _____

Insertion: _____

Innervation: _____

Blood Supply: _____

Function: _____

3. Obturator Internus

Origin: _____

Insertion: _____

Innervation: _____

Blood Supply: _____

Function: _____

4. Inferior Gemellus

Origin: _____

Insertion: _____

Innervation: _____

Blood Supply: _____

Function: _____

5. Quadratus Femoris

Origin: _____

Insertion: _____

Innervation: _____

Blood Supply: _____

Function: _____

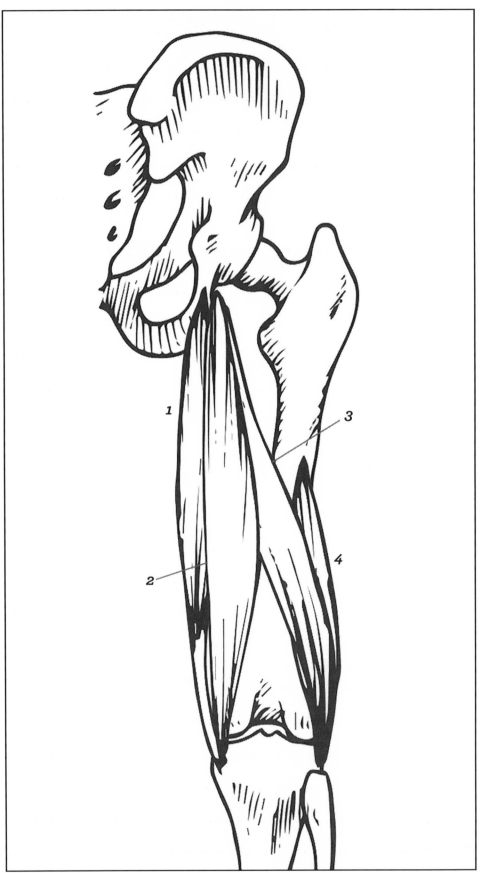

1. Semitendinosus

Origin: _____

Insertion: _____

Innervation: _____

Blood Supply: _____

Function: _____

2. Semimembranosus

Origin: _____

Insertion: _____

Innervation: _____

Blood Supply: _____

Function: _____

3. Biceps Femoris- Long Head

Origin: _____

Insertion: _____

Innervation: _____

Blood Supply: _____

Function: _____

4. Biceps Femoris- Short Head

Origin: _____

Insertion: _____

Innervation: _____

Blood Supply: _____

Function: _____

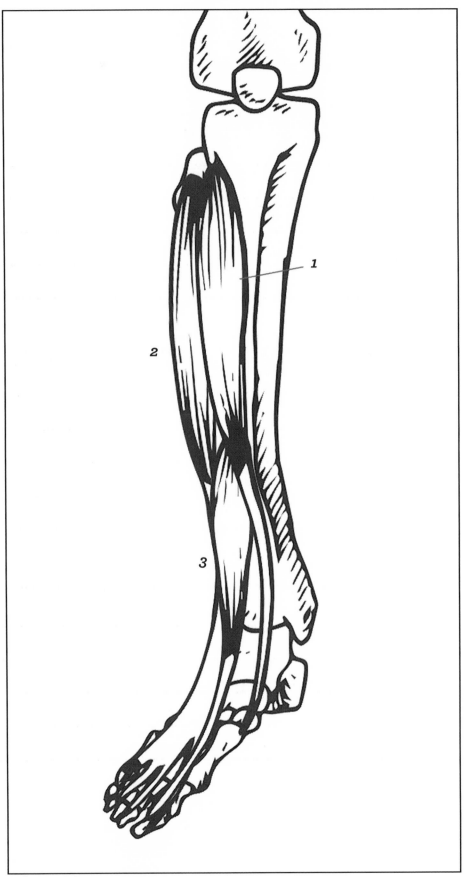

1. Tibialis Anterior

Origin: _____

Insertion: _____

Innervation: _____

Blood Supply: _____

Function: _____

2. Extensor Digitorum Longus

Origin: _____

Insertion: _____

Innervation: _____

Blood Supply: _____

Function: _____

3. Extensor Hallucis Longus

Origin: _____

Insertion: _____

Innervation: _____

Blood Supply: _____

Function: _____

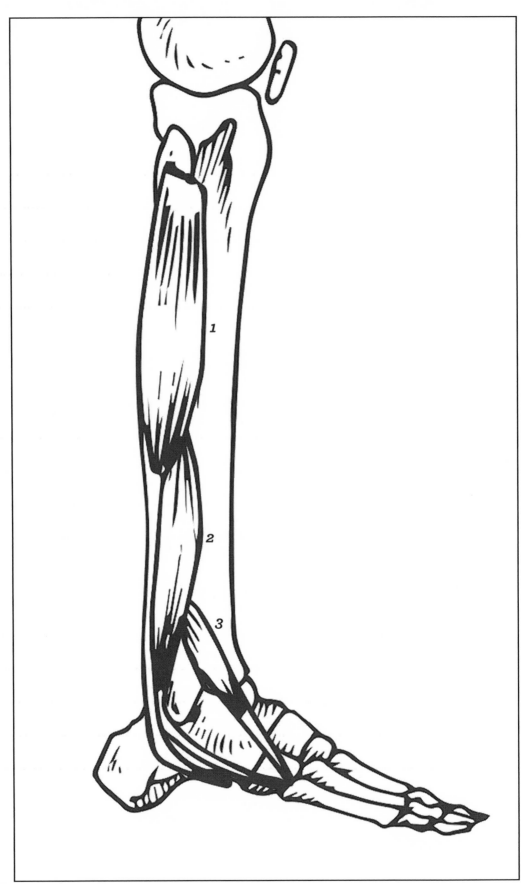

□ 1. Peroneus Longus

Origin: _____

Insertion: _____

Innervation: _____

Blood Supply: _____

Function: _____

□ 2. Peroneus Brevis

Origin: _____

Insertion: _____

Innervation: _____

Blood Supply: _____

Function: _____

□ 3. Peroneus Tertius

Origin: _____

Insertion: _____

Innervation: _____

Blood Supply: _____

Function: _____

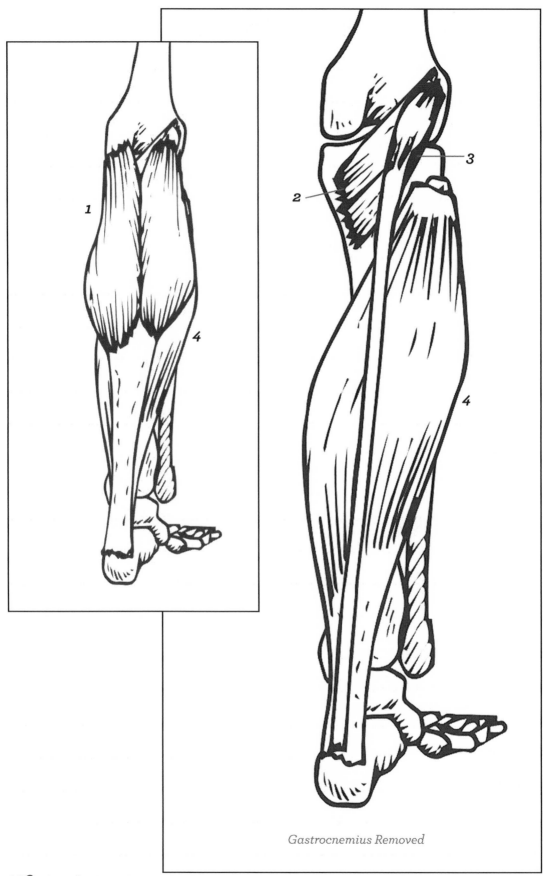

Gastrocnemius Removed

1. Gastrocnemius

Origin: _____

Insertion: _____

Innervation: _____

Blood Supply: _____

Function: _____

2. Popliteus

Origin: _____

Insertion: _____

Innervation: _____

Blood Supply: _____

Function: _____

3. Plantaris

Origin: _____

Insertion: _____

Innervation: _____

Blood Supply: _____

Function: _____

4. Soleus

Origin: _____

Insertion: _____

Innervation: _____

Blood Supply: _____

Function: _____

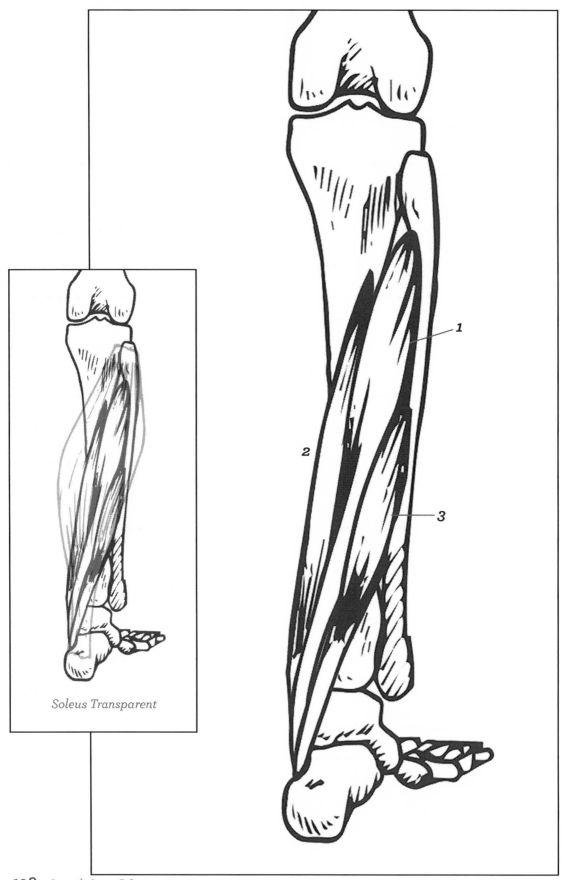

Soleus Transparent

1. Tibialis Posterior

Origin: _____

Insertion: _____

Innervation: _____

Blood Supply: _____

Function: _____

2. Flexor Digitorum Longus

Origin: _____

Insertion: _____

Innervation: _____

Blood Supply: _____

Function: _____

3. Flexor Hallucis Longus

Origin: _____

Insertion: _____

Innervation: _____

Blood Supply: _____

Function: _____

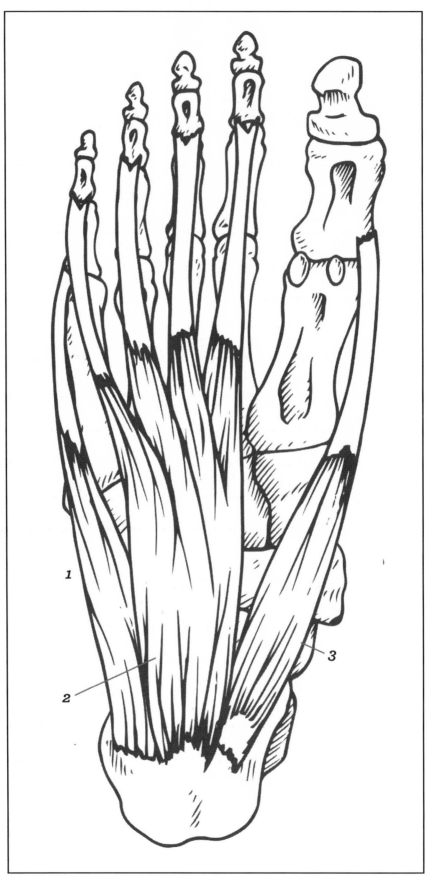

1. Abductor Digiti Minimi

Origin: _____

Insertion: _____

Innervation: _____

Blood Supply: _____

Function: _____

2. Flexor Digitorum Brevis

Origin: _____

Insertion: _____

Innervation: _____

Blood Supply: _____

Function: _____

3. Abductor Hallucis

Origin: _____

Insertion: _____

Innervation: _____

Blood Supply: _____

Function: _____

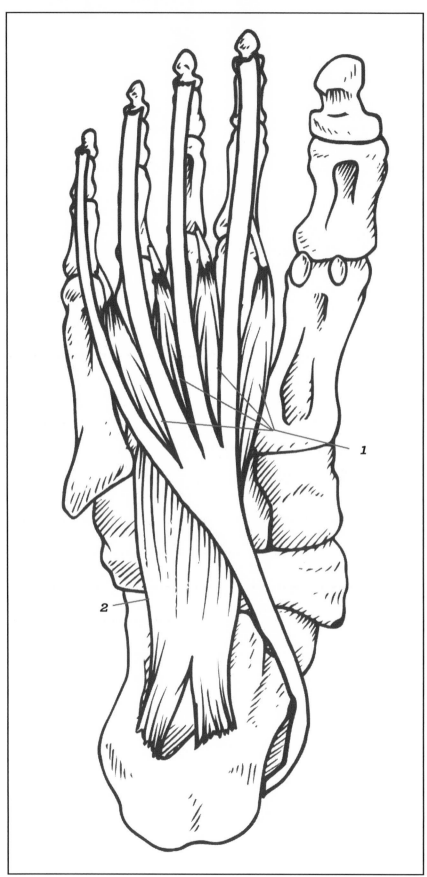

1

2

1. Lumbricals

Origin: _____

Insertion: _____

Innervation: _____

Blood Supply: _____

Function: _____

2. Quadrate Plantae

Origin: _____

Insertion: _____

Innervation: _____

Blood Supply: _____

Function: _____

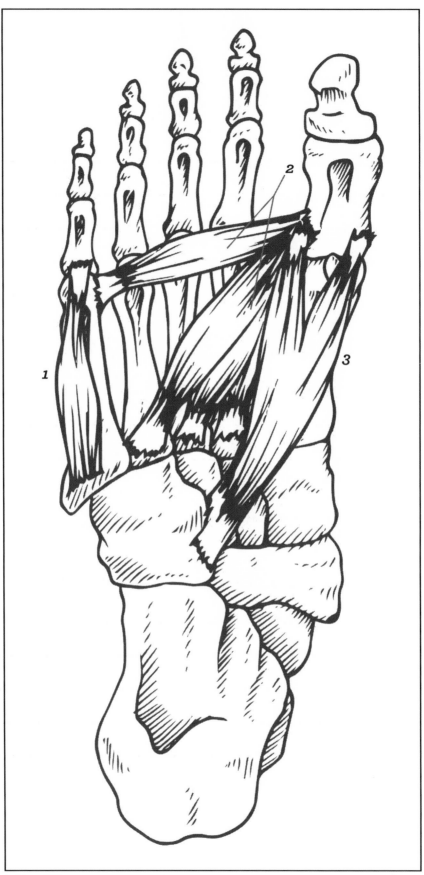

1. Flexor Digiti Minimi

Origin: _____

Insertion: _____

Innervation: _____

Blood Supply: _____

Function: _____

2. Adductor Hallucis

Origin: _____

Insertion: _____

Innervation: _____

Blood Supply: _____

Function: _____

3. Flexor Hallucis Brevis

Origin: _____

Insertion: _____

Innervation: _____

Blood Supply: _____

Function: _____

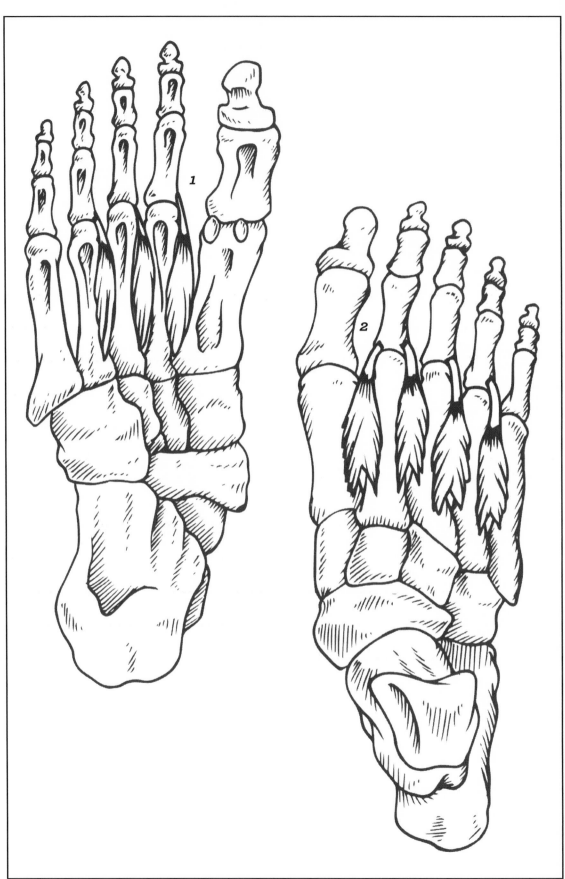

1. Plantar Interossei

Origin: _____

Insertion: _____

Innervation: _____

Blood Supply: _____

Function: _____

2. Dorsal Interossei

Origin: _____

Insertion: _____

Innervation: _____

Blood Supply: _____

Function: _____

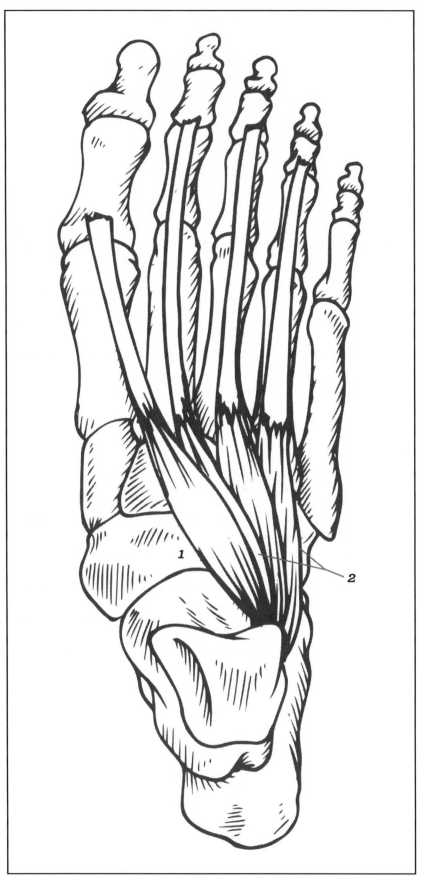

□ 1. Extensor Hallucis Brevis

Origin: _____

Insertion: _____

Innervation: _____

Blood Supply: _____

Function: _____

□ 2. Extensor Digitorum Brevis

Origin: _____

Insertion: _____

Innervation: _____

Blood Supply: _____

Function: _____

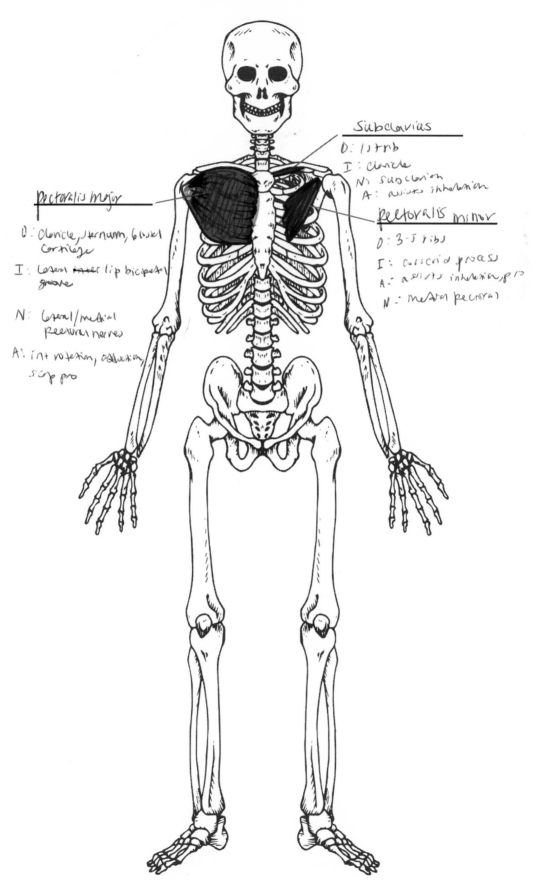

Subclavius
O: 1st rib
I: Clavicle
N: subclavian
A: assists inhalation

Pectoralis Major

O: Clavicle, sternum, bristol
Cartilage

I: Lateral inter lip bicipital
groove

N: lateral/medial
Pectoral nerves

A: int rotation, adduction
scap pro

Pectoralis minor

O: 3-5 ribs
I: coracoid process
A: assists inhalation, p ro
N: medial pectoral

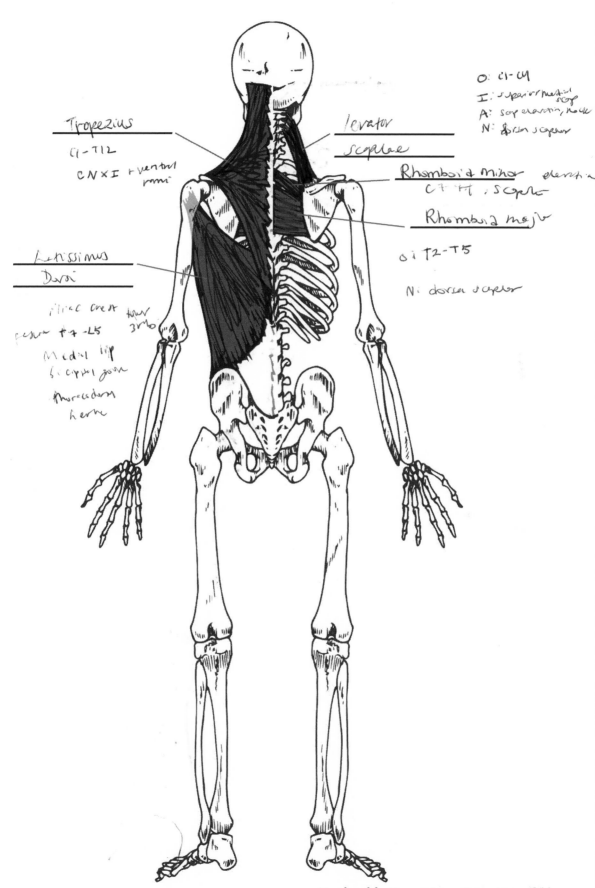

Trapezius
C1 - T12
CN XI + ventral rami

Levator
Scapulae

Rhomboid Minor   elevation
C7 + T1 : Scapula

Rhomboid Major
O: T2 - T5
N: dorsal scapular

O: C1 - C4
I: superior medial scap
A: scap elevation, rotate
N: dorsal scapular

Latissimus
Dorsi
iliac crest
fascia T7 - L5
Medial lip
bicipital groove
thoracodorsal
nerve
lower
3 ribs

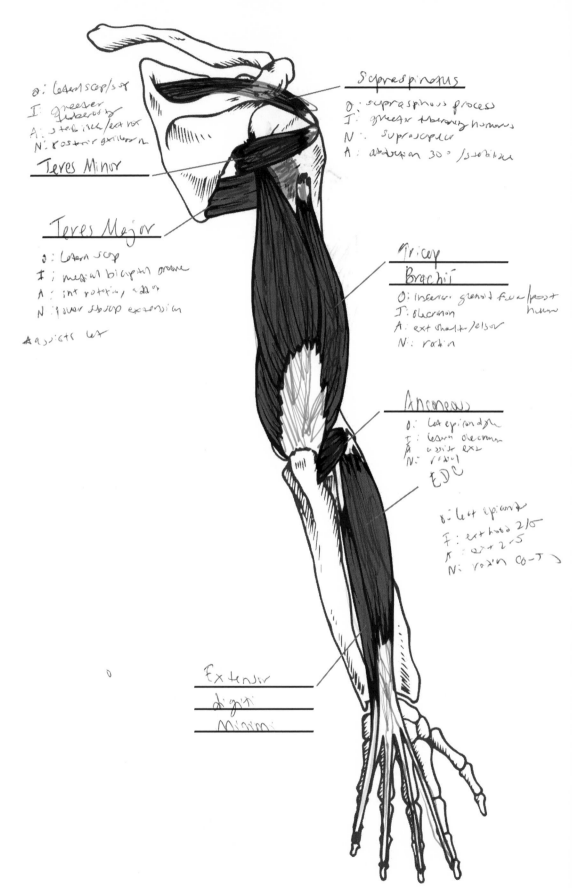

O: lateral scap/spr
I: greater
   tuberosity
A: lat tab incl/ext rot
N: rostral extension

Teres Minor

Suprespinatus

O: suprespinous process
I: greater throwing humerus
N: suprascapular
A: abduction 30° / stabilize

Teres Major

O: lateral scap
I: medial bicipital groove
A: int rotation, addon
N: lower subscap extension

Assists lat

Tricep
Brachii

O: inferior glenoid fascia/post
I: olecranon   hum
A: ext shoulder/elbow
N: radial

Anconeus

O: lat epicondyle
I: lateral olecranon
A: assist ext
N: radial

EDC

O: lat epicond
F: ext hood 2/5
A: ext 2-5
N: radial C6-7

Extensor

digiti

Minimi

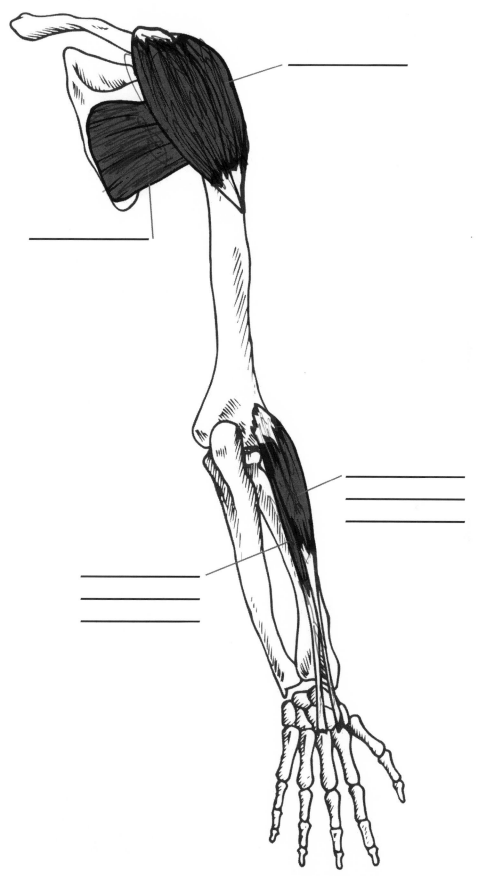

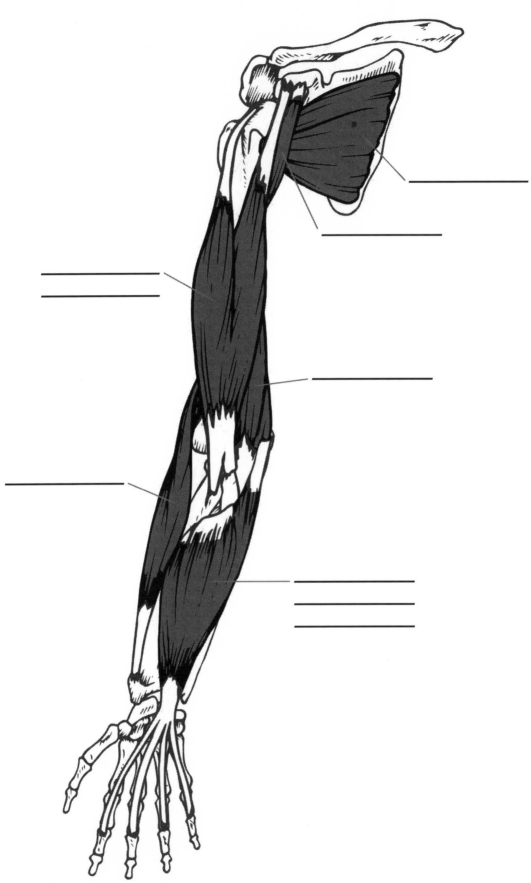

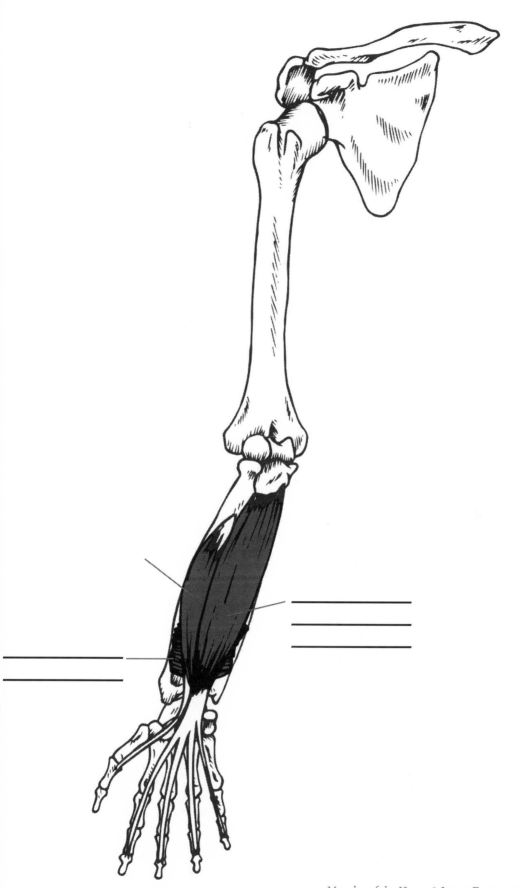

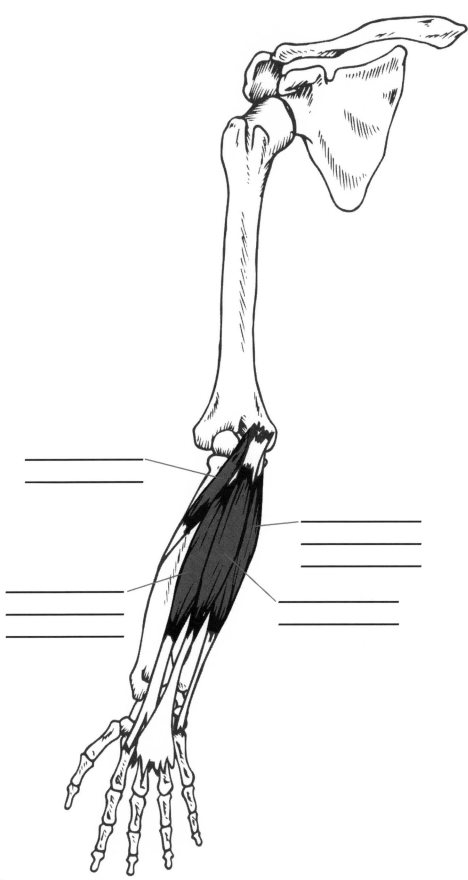

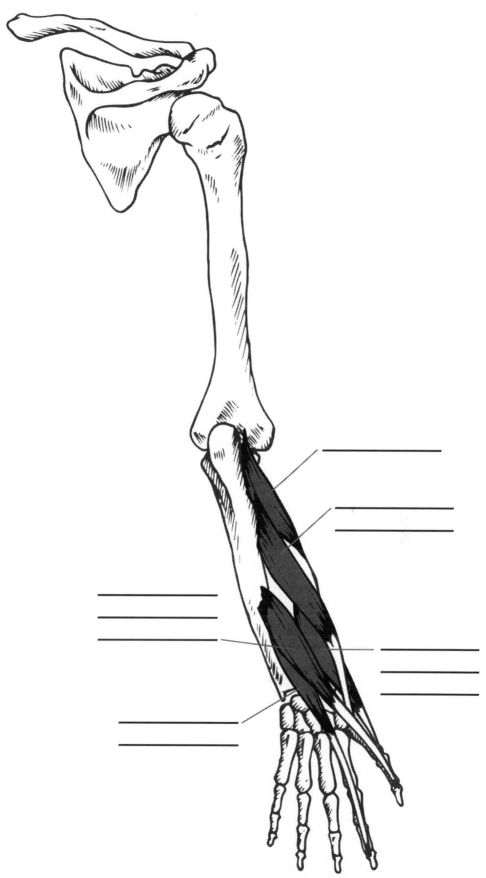

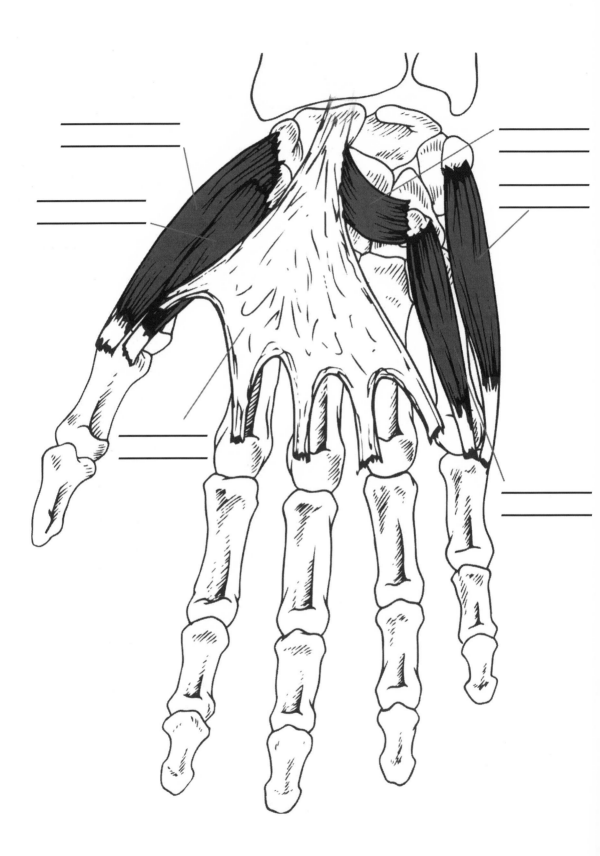

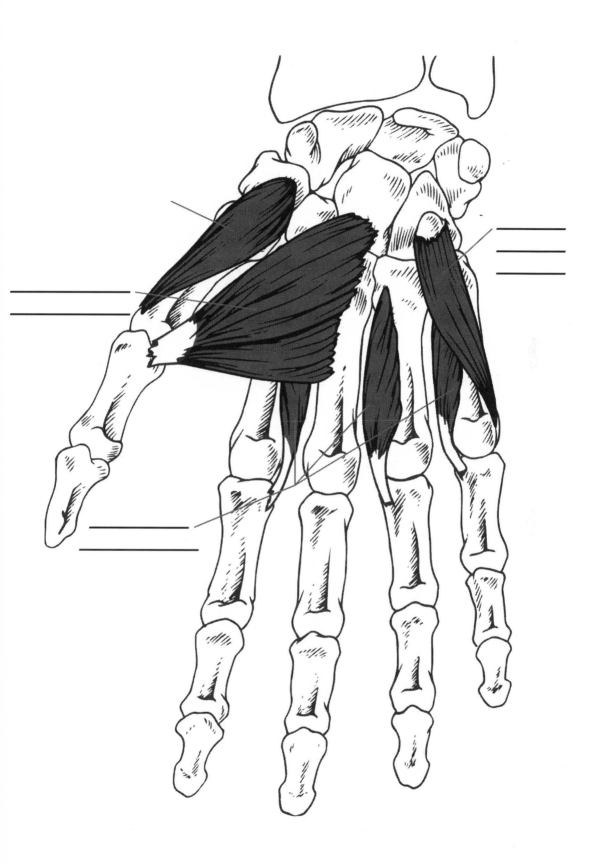

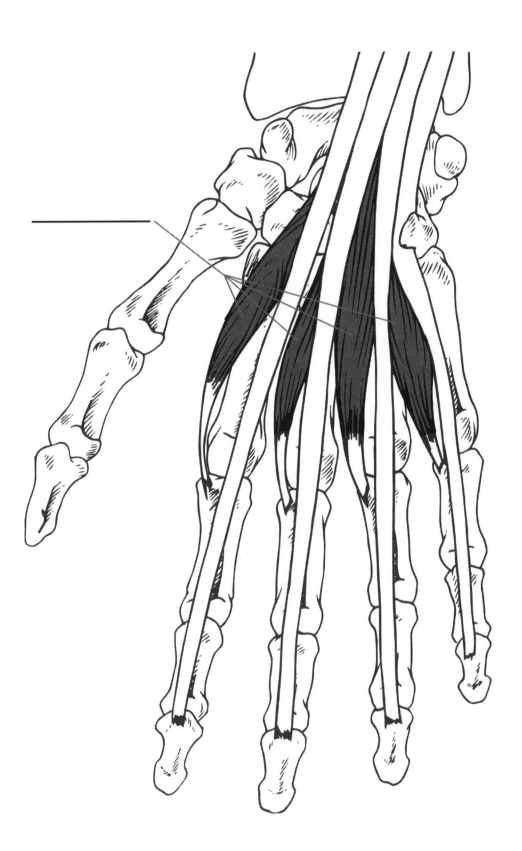

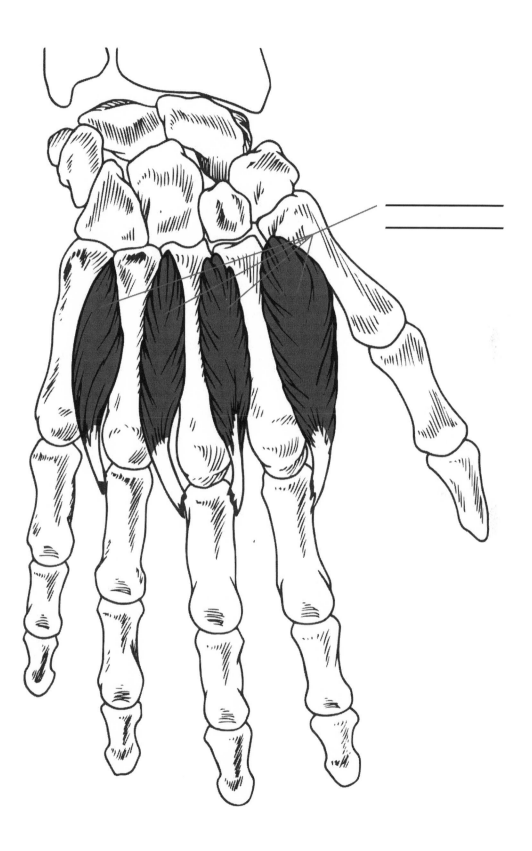

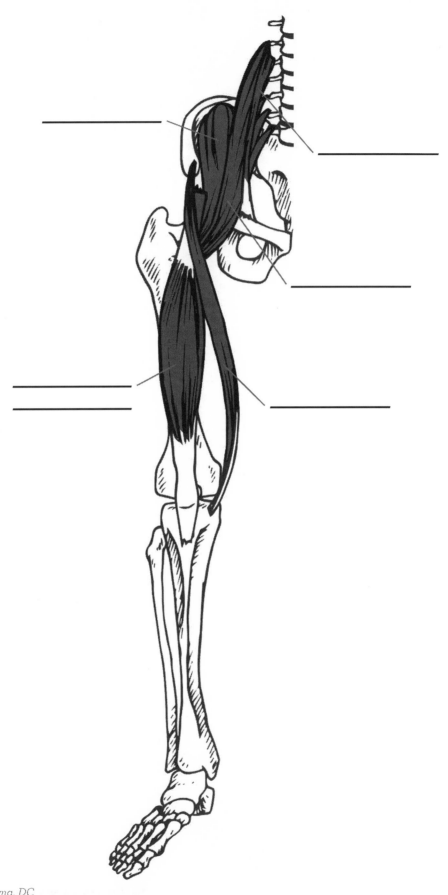

Sean de Lima, DC

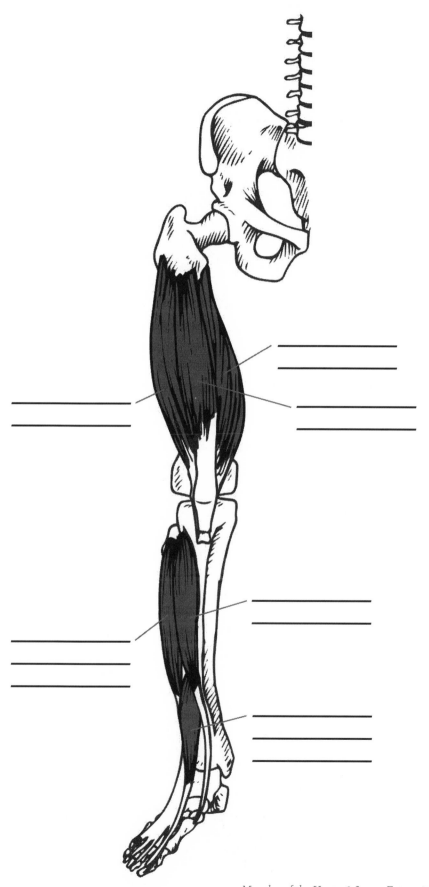

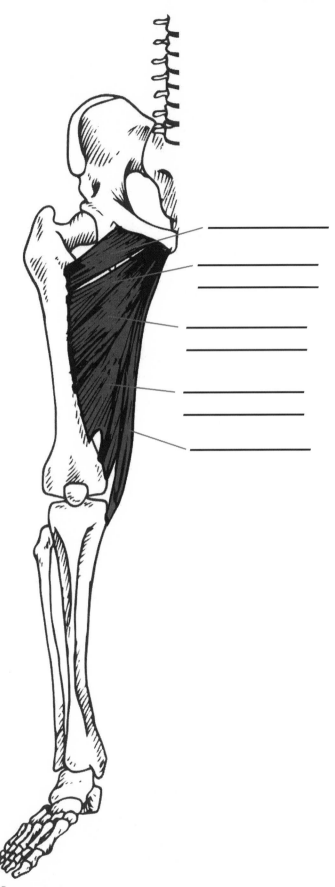

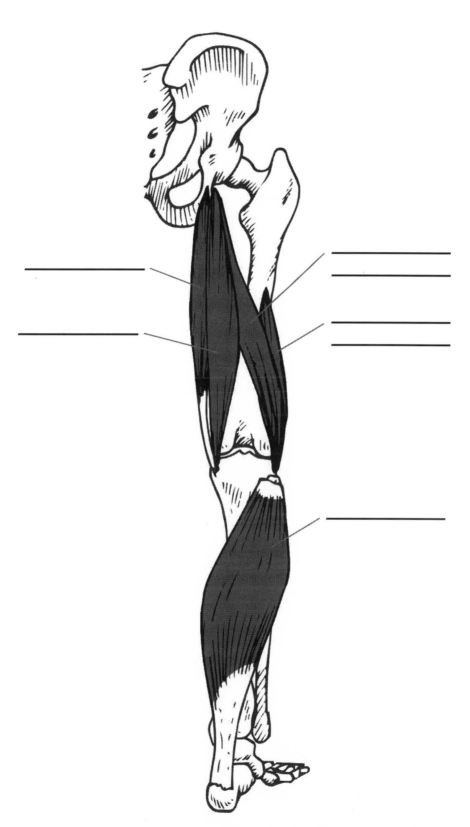

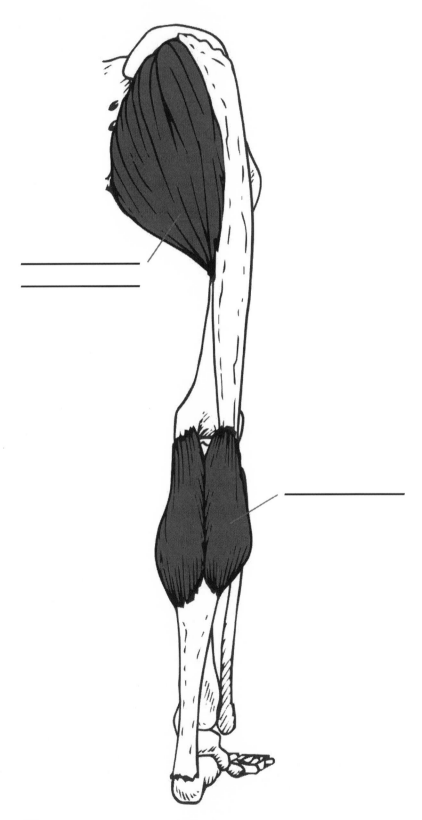

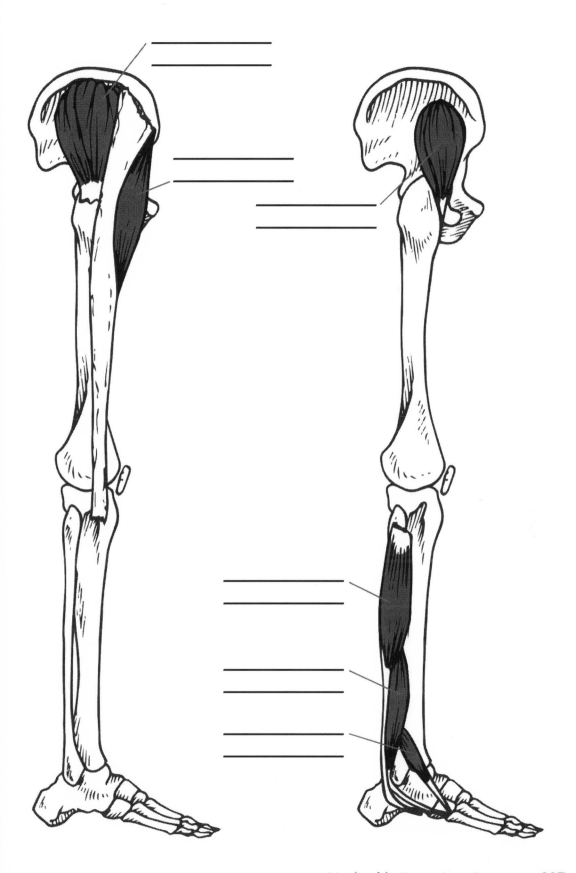

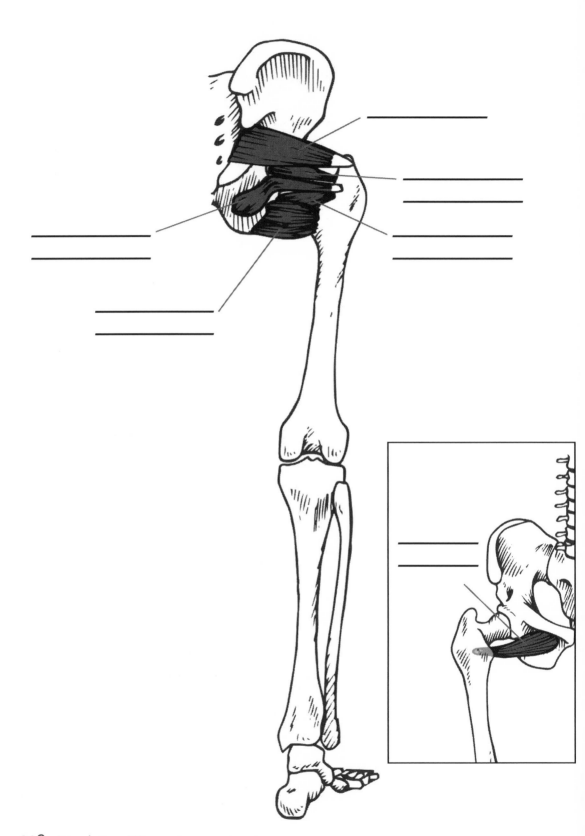

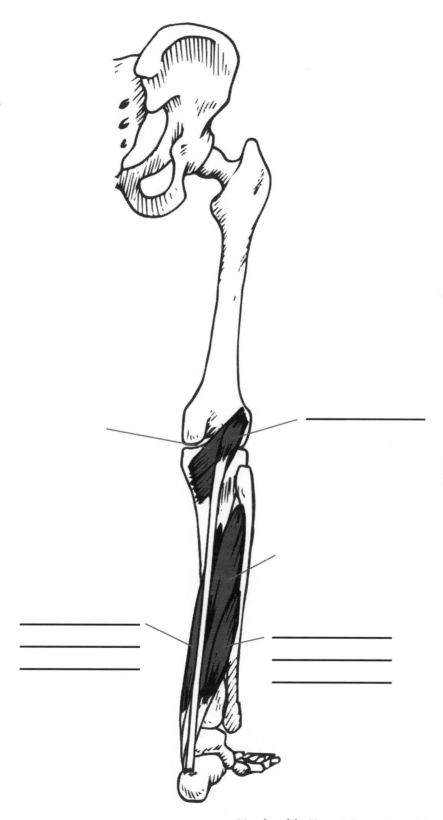

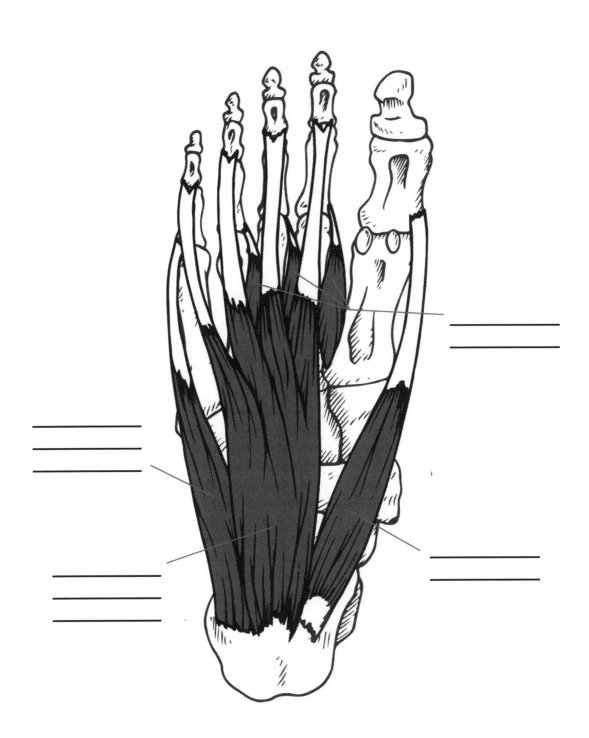

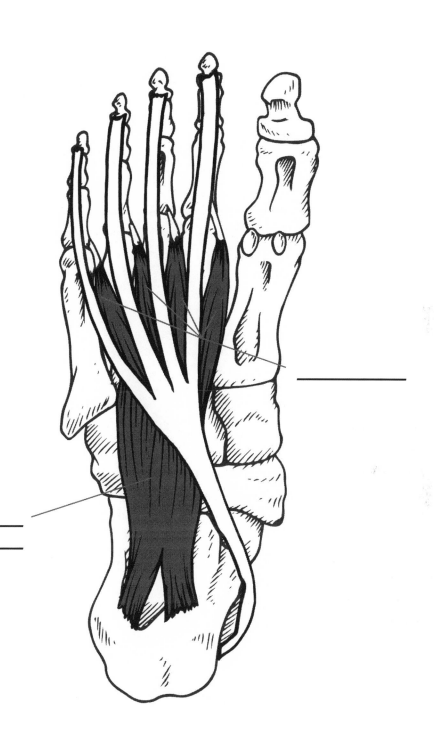

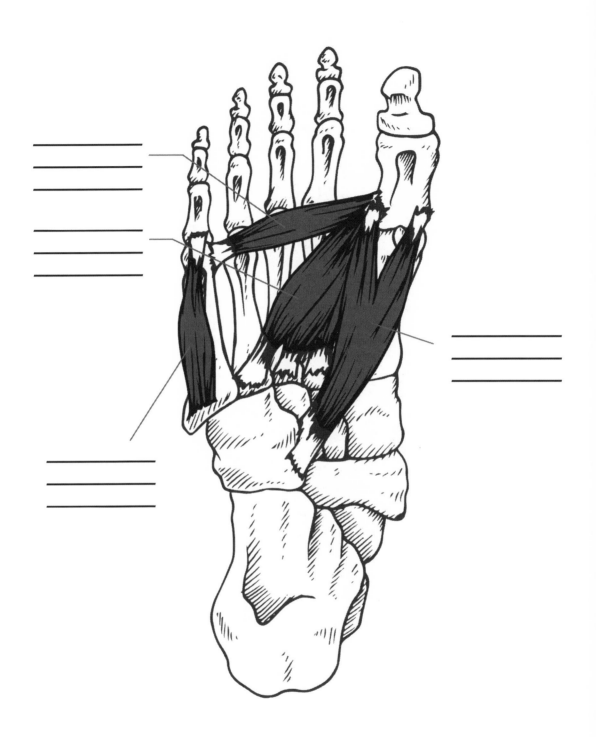

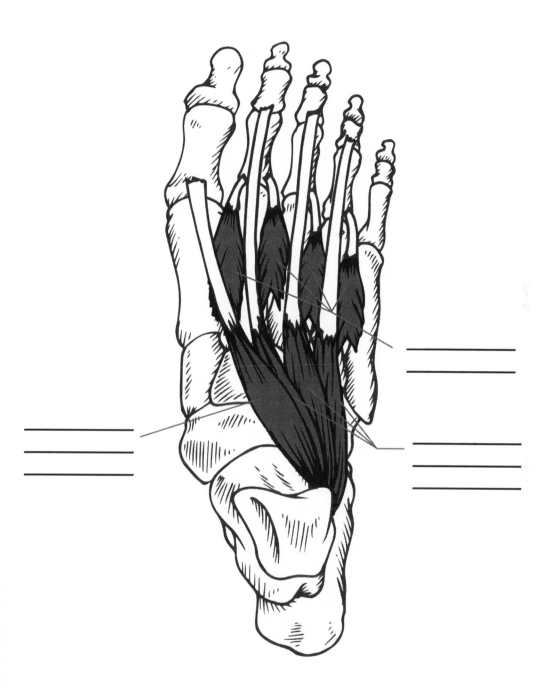

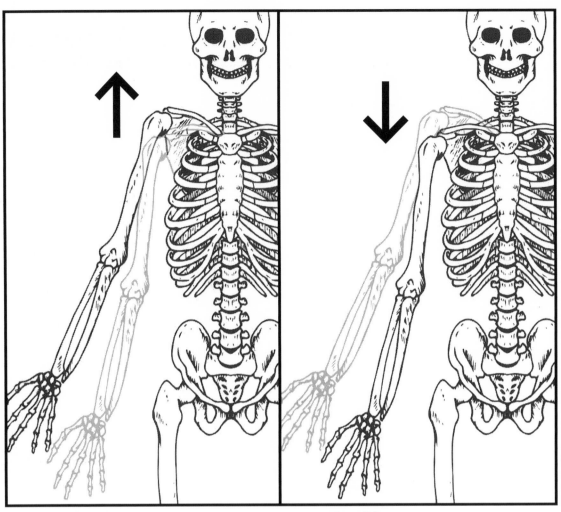

Shoulder: _____   *Shoulder:* _____

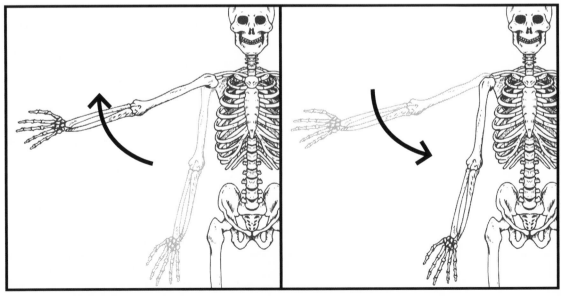

Arm: _____   *Arm:* _____

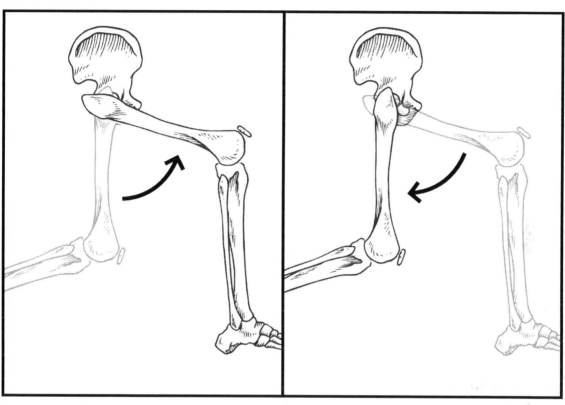

Hip: _____   *Hip:* _____

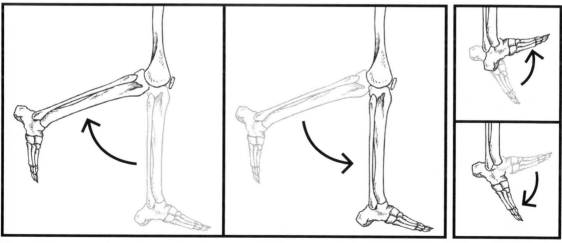

Knee: _____   *Knee:* _____

Foot:
_____ *Flexion /*
_____ *Flexion*

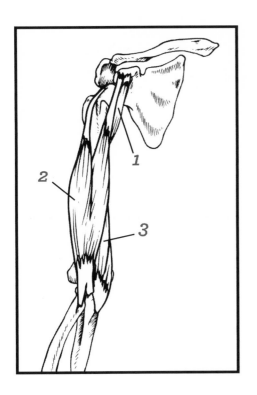

Muscles of the Musculocutaneous Nerve

1. _____

2. _____

3. _____

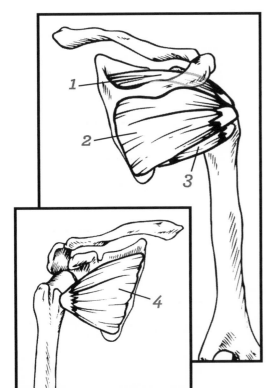

Muscles of the Rotator Cuff (S.I.T.S)

1. _____

2. _____

3. _____

4. _____

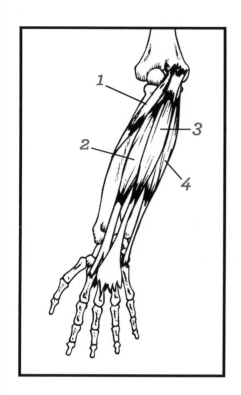

Muscles of the Common Flexor Tendon

1. _____

2. _____

3. _____

4. _____

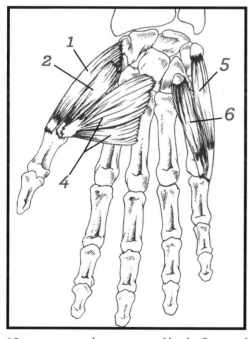

Thenar & Subthenar Muscles

1. _____

2. _____

3. *Opponens Pollicis**

4. _____

5. _____

6. _____

7. *Opponens Digiti Minimi**

*Opponens muscles are covered by the flexors of
the thumb and pinky*

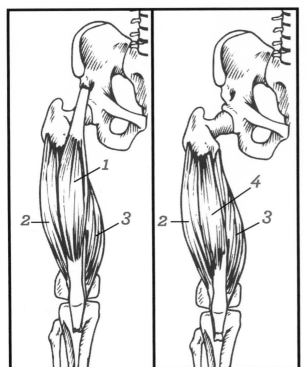

Muscles of the Quadriceps

1. _____

2. _____

3. _____

4. _____ *

*Vastus Intermedius is directly under Rectus Femoris

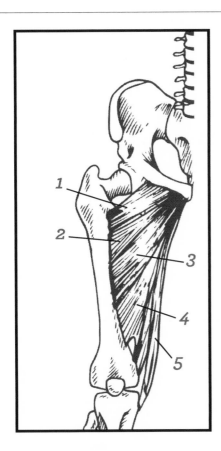

Adductor Muscles of the Thigh

1. _____

2. _____

3. _____

4. _____

5. _____

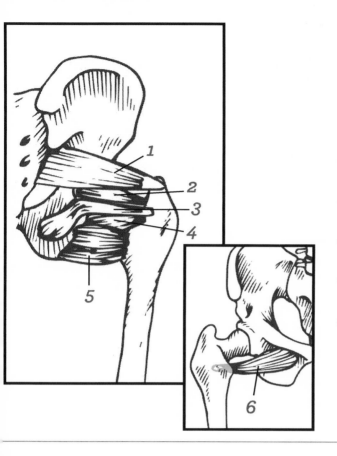

External Rotators of the Hip

1. _____

2. _____

3. _____

4. _____

5. _____

6. _____

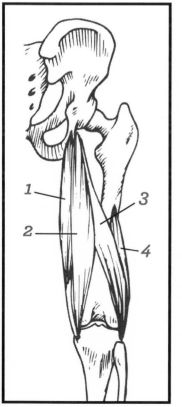

Hamstring Muscles

1. _____

2. _____

3. _____

4. _____

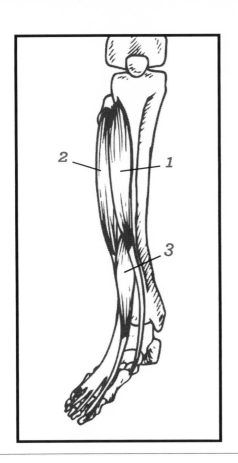

Anterior Compartment of the Leg

1. _____

2. _____

3. _____

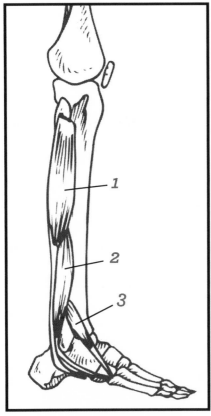

Lateral Compartment of the Leg

1. _____

2. _____

3. _____

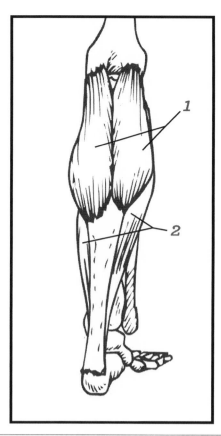

Posterior Compartment
of the Leg

1. _____

2. _____

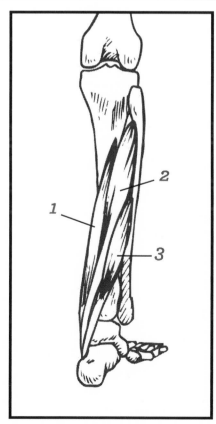

Medial Compartment
of the Leg

1. _____

2. _____

3. _____

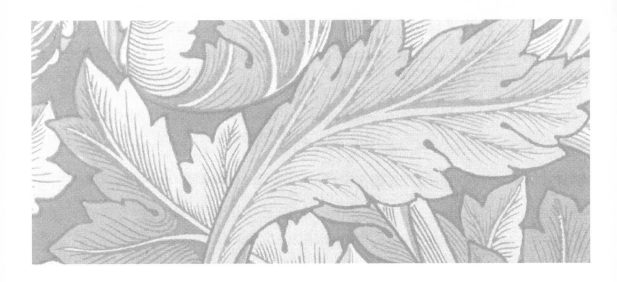

This is your chance to master your understanding
of how each muscle connects to the body. Grab a pencil and draw the
muscle directly onto the page! You don't need to be an artist to benefit from this.
By drawing, you are learning visually and kinesthetically at the same time.
Feel free to get creative. The following pages are meant to filled with notes, doodles,
scibbles, colors, anything that might help you to beter remember these muscles!

If you run out of space here, visit www.corticalmedia.com
to find printable pages to continue drawing.

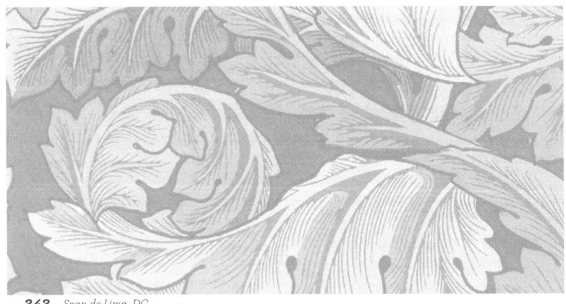

PART III:
Draw it Yourself

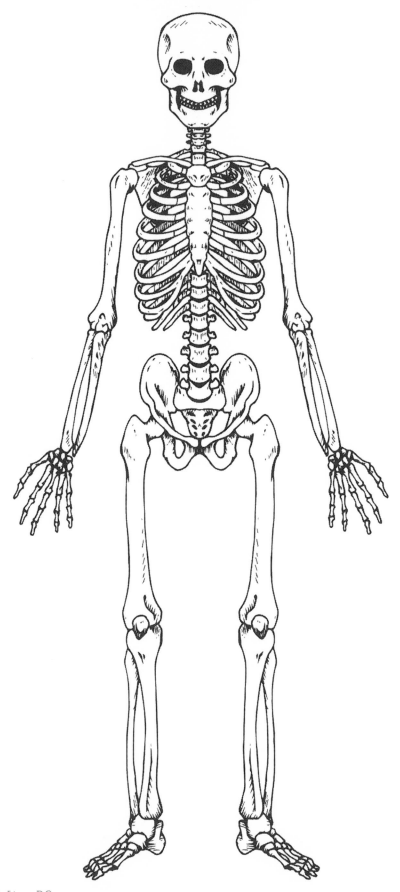

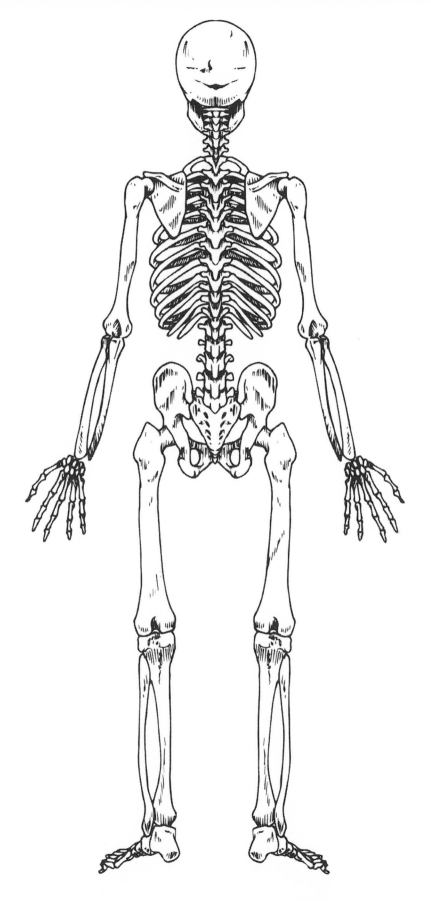

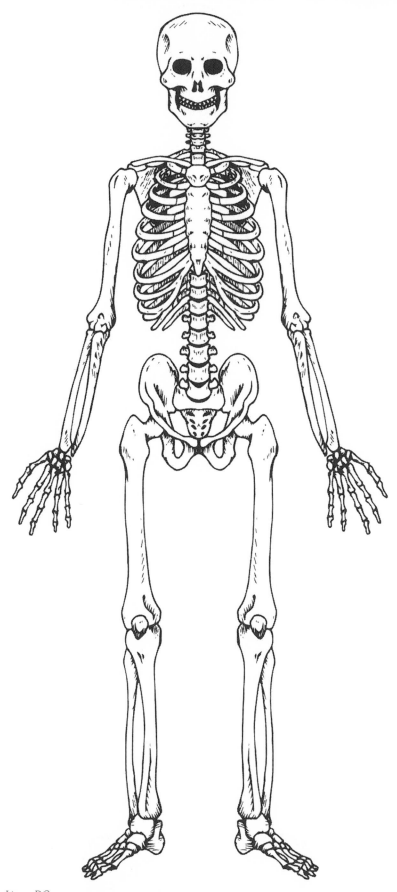

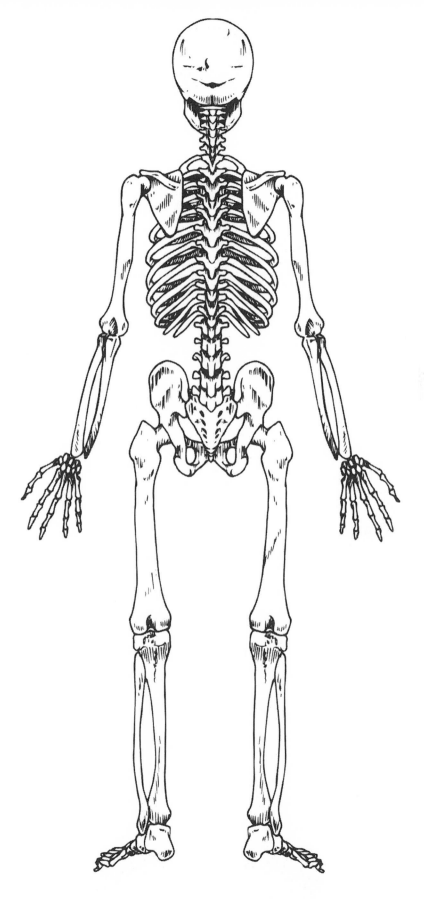

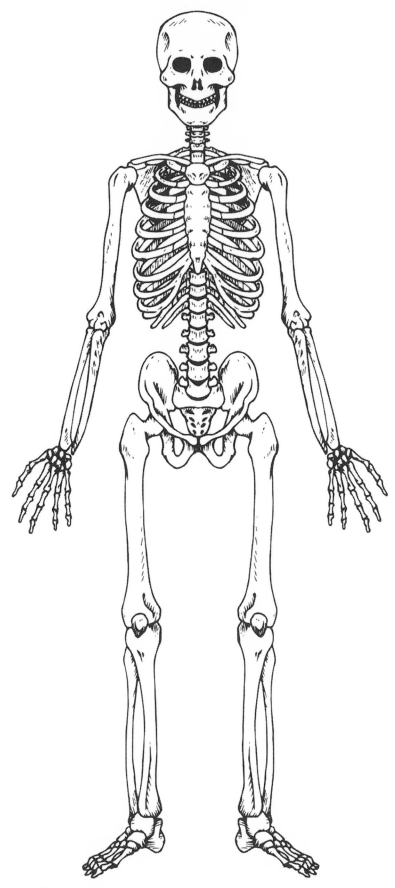

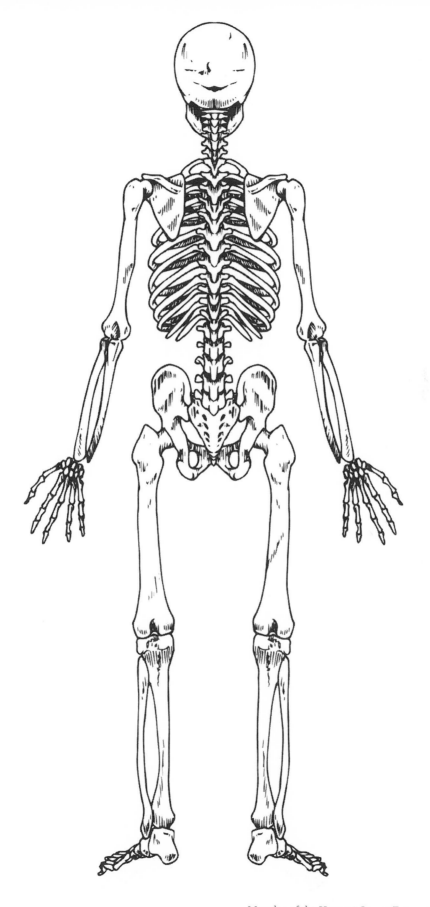

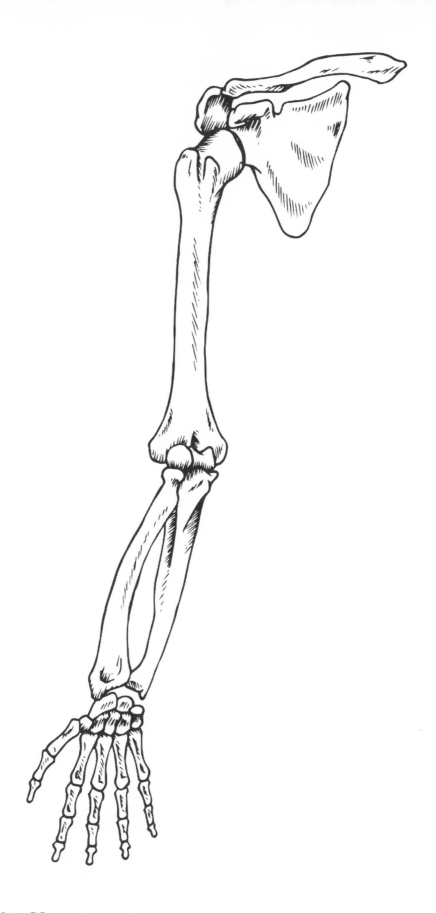

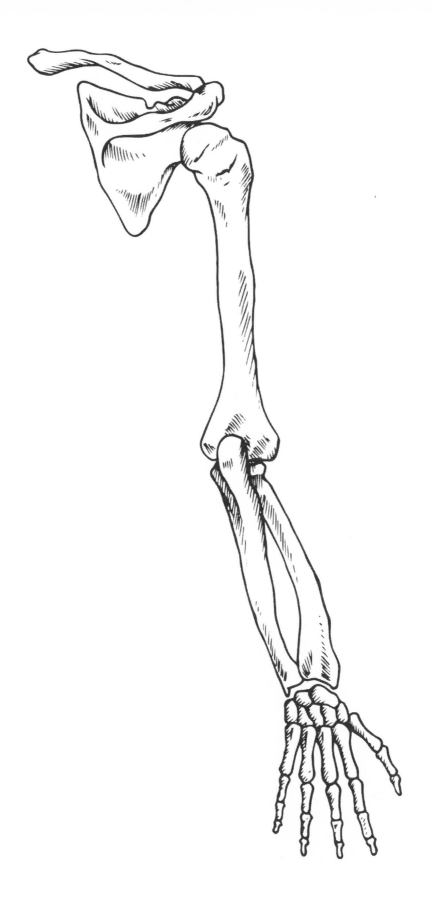

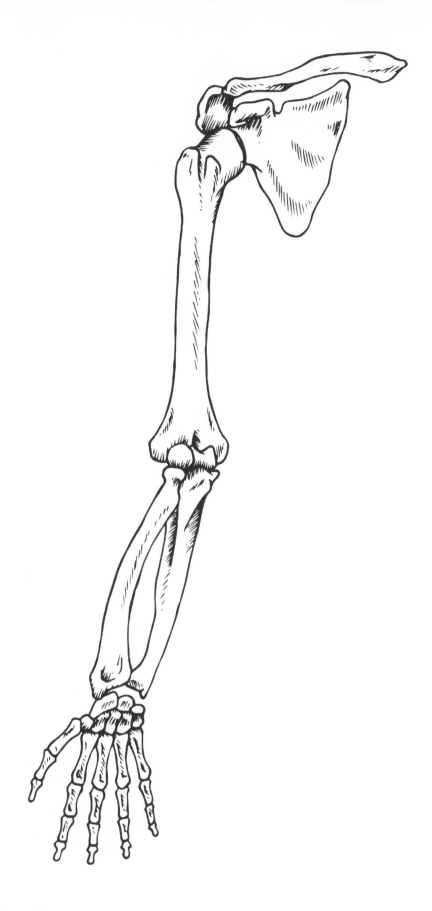

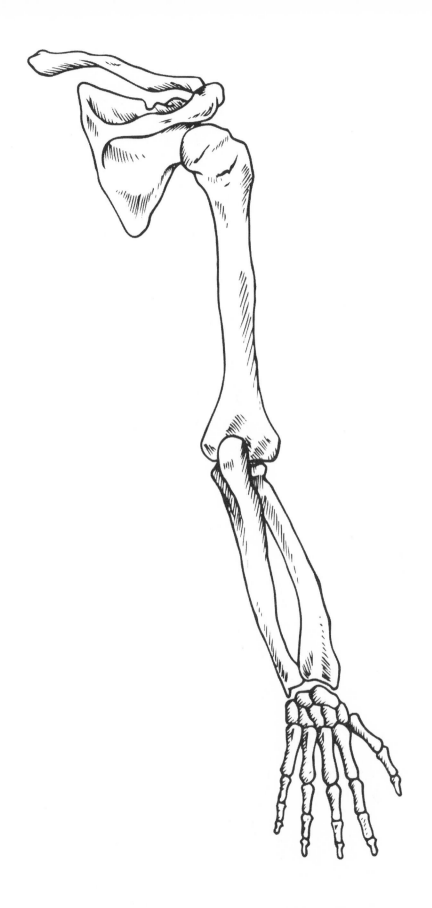

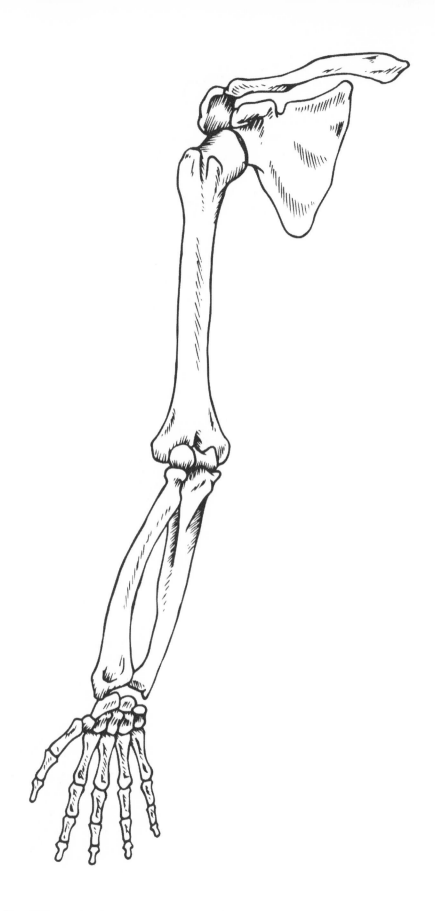

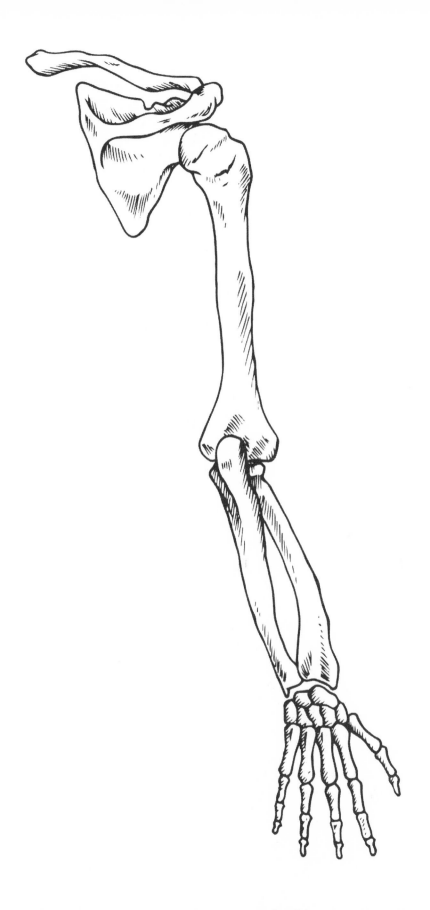

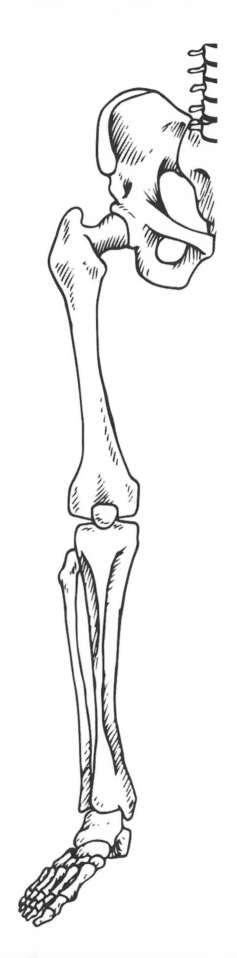

Sean de Lima, DC

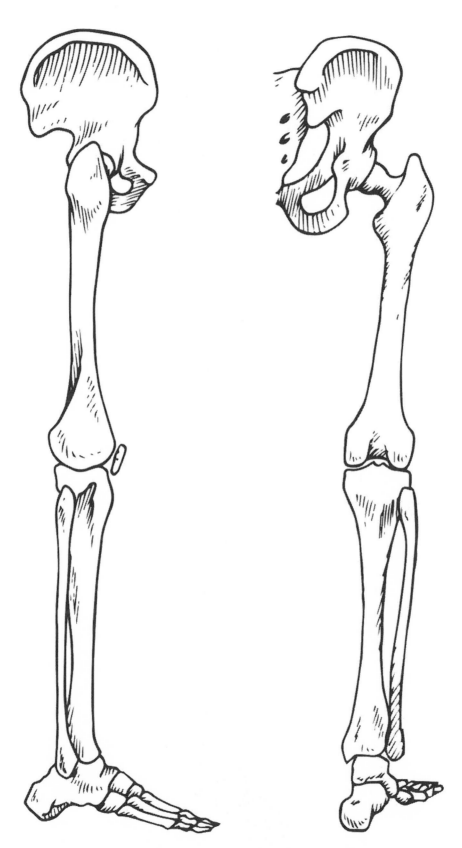

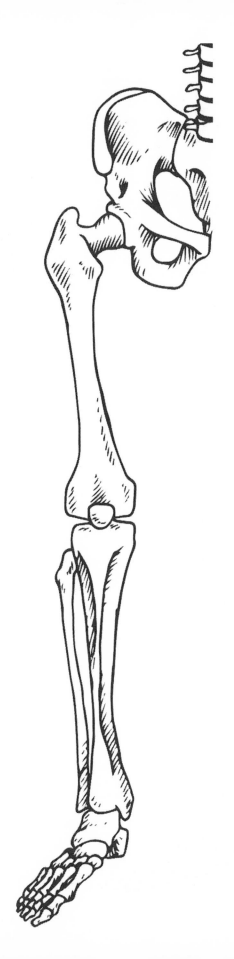

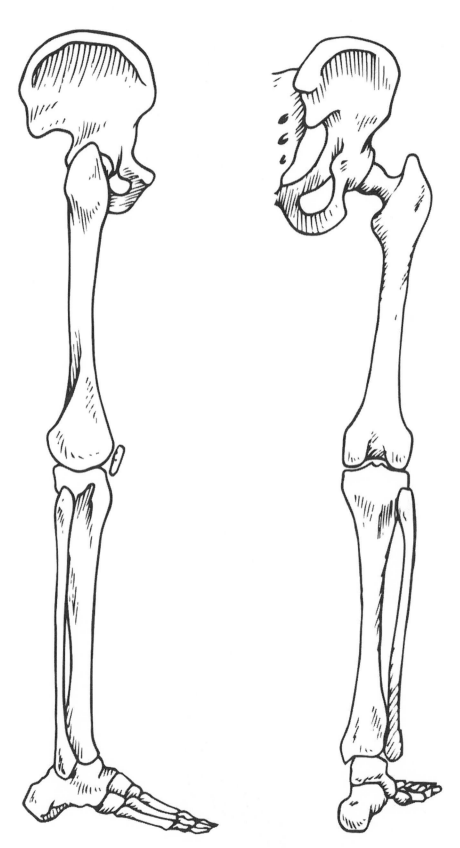

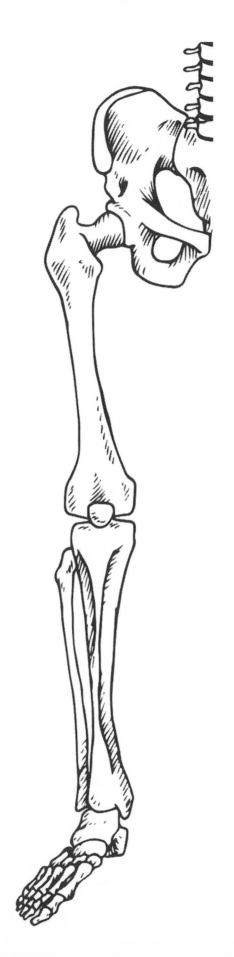

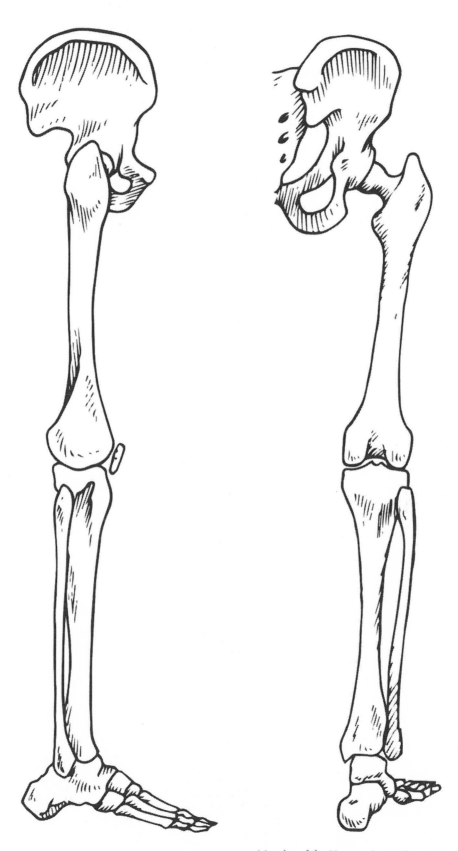

INDEX

INDEX

ABOUT THE AUTHOR

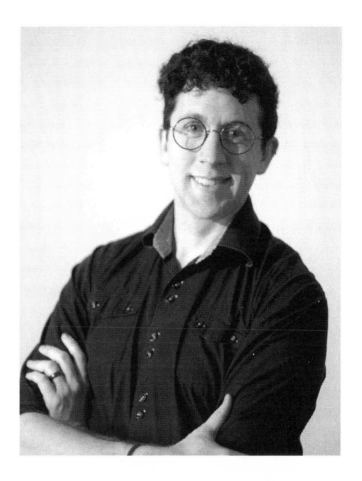

Sean de Lima completed his Doctorate of Chiropractic at Life Chiropractic College West in 2019. He practices in Calgary, Alberta where he lives with his husband and dogs.

This is Sean's first anatomy workbook. He has written and illustrated two children's storybooks.

Look for more of Sean's work at
www.corticalmedia.com

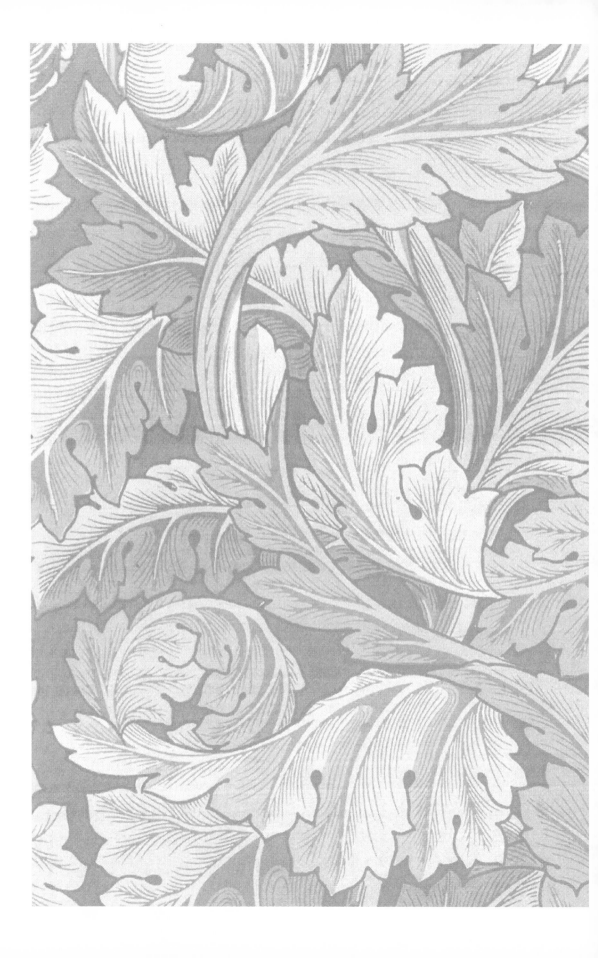

EDUCATIONAL INSTITUTIONS
Interested in using Anatomy Companion illustrations for in-class lectures?

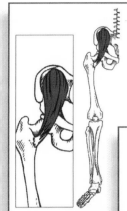
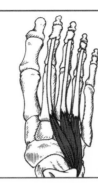
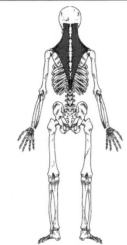
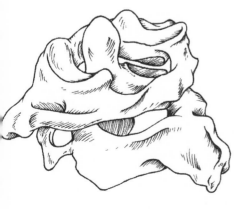

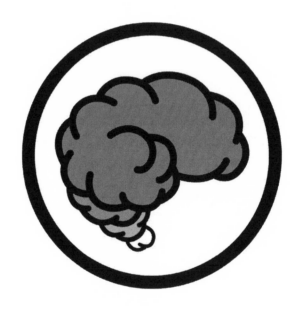

www.corticalmedia.com

Made in the USA
Middletown, DE
15 October 2020

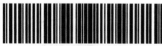